Intervention in Language Arts

A Practical Guide for Speech-Language Pathologists

By Kathryn P. DeKemel, Ph.D., CCC-SLP

Speech-Language Pathologist
Assistant Clinical Professor
Texas Women's University
Denton, Texas

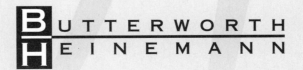
BUTTERWORTH
HEINEMANN

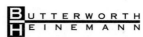

An Imprint of Elsevier Science

625 Walnut Street
Philadelphia, PA 19106

Intervention in Language Arts: A Practical Guide for Speech-Language Pathologists   ISBN 0-7506-7320-6

NOTICE

Speech-pathology is an ever-changing field. Standard safety precautions must be followed, but as new research and clinical experience broaden our knowledge, changes in treatment and drug therapy may become necessary or appropriate. Readers are advised to check the most current product information provided by the manufacturer of each drug to be administered to verify the recommended dose, the method and duration of administration, and contraindications. It is the responsibility of the licensed prescriber, relying on experience and knowledge of the patient, to determine dosages and the best treatment for each individual patient. Neither the publisher nor the author assumes any liability for any injury and/or damage to persons or property arising from this publication.

Library of Congress Cataloging-in-Publication Data
DeKemel, Kathryn P. (Kathryn Patrice)
   Intervention in language arts: a practical guide for the speech-language pathologist / by Kathryn P. Dekemel
     p. cm.
   Includes bibliographical references and index.
   ISBN 0-7506-7320-6
    1. Speech therapy—Study and teaching. 2. Speech therapy. 3. Language disorders—Treatment. I. Title.

RC428.D455 2003
616.85'506—dc21   2003045196

Publishing Director: Linda L. Duncan
Acquisitions Editor: Kellie White
Developmental Editor: Jennifer Watrous
Publishing Services Manager: John Rogers
Project Manager: Doug Turner
Designer: Amy Buxton

Printed in the United States of America.
Last digit is the print number: 9   8   7   6   5   4   3   2   1

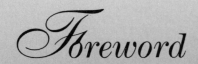

Foreword

. . . it may be far more productive to view language impairment (LI) in preschoolers not only for what it is at present, but also for what it is likely to become as the child grows older. (Fey, Catts, and Larrivee, 1995, p. 3)*

These provocative words written several years ago by Fey, Catts, and Larrivee (1995)* remind speech-language pathologists and other specialists who work with children and adolescents with language-learning problems that the road to success may be a long one. Indeed, most preschoolers with language disorders fail to outgrow them—a point made throughout the text. The beauty of *Intervention in Language Arts: A Practical Guide for Speech-Language Pathologists* is that it helps readers appreciate the ways in which language disorders change and evolve over time. The text helps professionals see what language impairment looks like at school-age levels, bringing the words of Fey and his colleagues to life. As a result, the text is a useful resource for professionals who are interested in both younger and older children.

The power of the text, in addition to covering the school-age area with depth and insight, is three-fold: (1) the text presents practical and useable suggestions for language intervention within strong theoretical frameworks; (2) the text includes numerous tables, checklists, and other supporting materials that bridge the theory-to-practice gap; and (3) the text provides examples of students' performances on a number of tasks, examples that contribute to its applicability.

*Fey, M. E., Catts, H. W., and Larrivee, L. S. (1995). Preparing preschoolers for the academic and social challenges of school. In M. E. Fey, J. Windsor, and S. F. Warren (Eds.), *Language intervention: Preschool through the elementary years* (pp. 3-37). Baltimore, MD: Paul H. Brookes.

Dr. DeKemel helps readers weave their way through the complex maze of what-to-do's with children and adolescents in trouble. The chapters are organized with an elegant and structurally coherent style. It might be said, to use a cliché, that the text practices what it preaches. The book is a metaphor for effective language intervention. For example, a clear purpose section introduces each chapter. The bullet-point approach prepares readers for the theoretical information that follows. This technique creates an explicit macrostructure for readers and sets the tone for the text, while at the same time facilitating readers' memory and comprehension, two areas of significant concern in language-learning–disabled students. Dr. Kemel's style helps readers access their background knowledge and prepare for information that might be less familiar to them. The intervention plans, questionnaires, and other supporting materials that are outlined in each chapter become semantic webs for professionals. Student samples complete the assessment and intervention road maps.

One never gets the feeling that the intervention suggestions presented come from thin air, outdated models, or the latest craze in language and literacy. Rather, the language intervention concepts are steeped in current research, data, and experience. The book begins with a strong conceptual framework. The discussion of memory, inferences, and the comprehension of narrative discourse puts the critical pieces of school-age language disorders in the forefront for readers. This choice, starting with the memory-inferencing-discourse topic, is daring. The discussion helps speech-language pathologists and other professionals appreciate the challenges facing them. However, the text never falls short by leaving readers feeling overwhelmed with theory. By contrast, Dr. DeKemel not only gives readers the hardened truth about the complexity of the behaviors they are trying to modify but she also provides some answers to the Where do I begin? and Where do I go? questions. Dr. DeKemel also reminds professionals early in the text that children often *have* processing/comprehension strategies but they may need specific help in learning how to apply them to specific tasks and situations. Again, this concept, along with others that readers will discover, encourages them to think outside of the proverbial intervention box. A number of connections, including the SLI (Specific Language Impairment)/LLD (language-learning disabilities) connection and the spoken/written language connection, are articulated coherently and accurately.

Like a pair of matched bookends, the beginning and ending chapters form a perfectly balanced package. Chapter 8 asks speech-language pathologists to consider a very hard reality: how long do I keep language-disordered children on my caseload (or in therapy)? Dealing with both the dismissal dilemma and the long-term follow-up of language-disordered students, to use Dr. DeKemel's words, are major challenges for practicing professionals. But again, as she has done throughout the text, Dr. DeKemel provides a number of excellent suggestions for her readers. Using results from a pilot study, she brings real world relevance to the intervention techniques offered. The tables in the chapter are rich in detail; they provide school-based speech and language professionals with guidelines that facilitate dismissal and follow-up decisions. The checklist that outlines the minimal language competencies by age and grade levels is especially useful and brings readers back to what Fey, Catts, and Larrivee (1995)* are talking about.

Between the first and last installments is a treasure chest of information. Although the text is geared toward speech-language pathologists, it should reach a wider audience. Regular and special educators, reading specialists, and other front-line professionals would find this text very helpful. A number of chapters cut across discipline-specific interests. The chapter on miscue analysis brings together a number of perspectives. It brings oral and written language closer together, presents a literate discussion of LLD subgroups, and provides suggestions for integrating quantitative and quali-

tative assessment results. The chapter also presents a systemic view of language form, content, and use. The samples of real students, with and without language and literacy problems, clarify points made. Clinicians and teachers will recognize the students in the profiles and, as a result, make better intervention choices. The intervention suggestions that are outlined for the heterogeneous group of students take readers as far away from a one-size-fits-all intervention approach as one can get.

Intervention in Language Arts asks its readers to reflect upon many aspects of school-age language disorders. The text takes a hard look at current practices and perceptions in the field of language, learning, and literacy. It brings the role of the speech-language pathologist into perspective in written language and creates bridges between what is known and what is new. For example, the chapter on spelling and writing asks speech-language pathologists to think about the terms *intelligibility* and *legibility* as a link between oral and written language concepts. There are jewels like this one throughout the text that make the information more meaningful for its audience. Readers are taken through a tremendous amount of material embedded in a structure that enables them to keep the forest in mind while considering its individual trees.

Several years ago there was a blue-jeans commercial that used the catch phrase "No excuses." For some reason the phrase found its way into my consciousness from long-term memory after reading this book. I cannot remember exactly why the line was used in the commercial, but I kept thinking about how fortunate we are to practice in an era that is rich in research, theoretical, and practical advances. As a school-based speech-language pathologist and professor/supervisor of graduate-level speech-language clinicians, I hear laments like "I don't know where to begin with my older language-disordered students," "I don't have the time to add written-language intervention to my already overwhelming caseload responsibilities," "I have to do spelling, too?", "He just doesn't remember what I teach him," and "I feel the pressure to keep all these students on my caseload." Although there is validity to many of these and related concerns, there are also "no excuses" for accepting cookbook solutions for complex problems. Research of the past 3 decades alone has provided

*Fey, M. E., Catts, H. W., and Larrivee, L. S. (1995). Preparing preschoolers for the academic and social challenges of school. In M. E. Fey, J. Windsor, and S. F. Warren (Eds.), *Language intervention: Preschool through the elementary years* (pp. 3-37). Baltimore, MD: Paul H. Brookes.

us with a rich knowledge base. We have come far from the days when we knew little about what happens to our preschoolers with language disorders and how to help them succeed academically and socially. Dr. DeKemel's *Intervention in Language Arts* reminds us that while the road may be a long one, the future is looking brighter for the LLD students in our care. Dr. DeKemel's text points us in a direction that speaks to the creation of innovative, integrated, and theoretically sound language intervention approaches.

Geraldine P. Wallach, Ph.D.
Associate Professor and Clinic Director
California State University, Long Beach
Department of Communicative Disorders
Long Beach, California
March 2003

Preface

During my 17 years as a practicing speech-language pathologist (SLP) and 9 years as a university instructor and clinical supervisor in the field of communication sciences and disorders (COMD), I have frequently heard both students and SLP colleagues complain about the paucity of therapy-based literature in our field. By *therapy-based literature*, I am not referring to the abundant manuals, picture stimuli cards, games, and other therapy-related materials of that nature so readily available from a variety of companies that one can browse through at the exhibit halls of conventions and conferences. Rather, I am referring to a lack of textbooks, journal articles, and other scholarly works that provide detailed and specific information on *how to do* therapy. More to the point, I am concerned that much of our professional literature fails to explore how *theory* is related to *therapy*, or put another way, how *research* is connected to *practice*. I am certainly not the only one to express this concern about this growing disconnect in our discipline. Our national organization has long lamented the lack of collaboration between researchers and practitioners, and plans are in motion to address this problem in a variety of ways (for instance, the new American Speech-Language-Hearing Association [ASHA] guidelines for academic and clinical training). Concerns about the disconnect as it relates to the training of graduate students remain extremely relevant. We have all probably had the unfortunate experience of being enrolled in a COMD course that provided a detailed discussion of theory (i.e., a definition of the communication disorder in question, its symptomatology, etiology, etc.) but rarely devoted equal time to treatment issues. The new ASHA guidelines stress that there must be a clear and strong link between academic coursework and the skills required in clinical practicum. Furthermore, COMD training programs must begin to measure students' mastery of core academic knowledge and basic clinical competencies in much the same way we measure outcomes in the real world. It is hoped

that these changes will alleviate the all-too-familiar problem of beginning clinicians entering the workforce who are, despite extensive training in graduate school, still deficient in some of the most basic clinical skills. Beginning clinicians often possess an abundant store of academic knowledge but are simply unable to translate that knowledge into practical clinical applications.

Another issue is that long after our formal university training ends and we find ourselves at conferences or conventions in the pursuit of continuing education units to maintain our licensure, SLPs are still often frustrated by the lack of continuing education sessions that deal specifically with treatment issues. It would appear that speech-language theory is something we are expected to learn formally in our profession, whereas how to do therapy is something we are expected to learn the hard way, by way of trial and error out in the trenches.

Ironically, changes during the 1990s and through the early 2000s in federal legislation that have affected both the provision of speech-language therapy services in schools and rehabilitation settings may actually be a blessing in disguise for our profession. As we are held increasingly accountable for documenting our clients' gains in treatment (in order to secure or maintain reimbursement for services), our professional organizations and state associations have responded with a call to action. This call to action has urged researchers to design and implement more treatment efficacy and outcome studies, as well as to have increased participation and collaboration of practicing clinicians with researchers on such efficacy and outcomes projects. It is hoped that this efficacy and outcomes research, along with participation from SLPs out in the field, will help to bridge the gap between research and practice that has existed for decades in our profession.

It was this very call to action and a desire to successfully blend theory and practice in the field of COMD that prompted me write this book. This is a book designed for practicing SLP clinicians, graduate clinicians in training, and related service professionals in fields such as psychology, regular education, and special education who deal with language-learning–disabled (LLD) students in school settings. The book explores the latest research findings in the area of spoken and written language deficits (note that the boundaries between these domains is increasingly disappearing) and examines how those new research findings are radically altering both theory and practice. Specific attention is paid to the why and how of intervention for these disorders. I address the following important question: How can SLPs, who traditionally have *not* had extensive exposure to the areas of reading and writing in their graduate curriculum, address these problems in a holistic fashion that will benefit students both communicatively and academically?

I advocate a holistic approach to diagnosis, assessment, and treatment of language-learning disabilities, whereby the SLP functions as a dynamic member of a multidisciplinary team, consisting of regular and special education teachers, parents, administrators, and other related service providers. Attention is focused on the fact that SLPs no longer provide services solely in small therapy rooms in the schools (i.e., the traditional pull-out therapy model). Indeed, we are increasingly functioning as communication teachers or language specialists for the entire school, entering classrooms and collaborating with classroom teachers to address a variety of linguistic and communication-related concerns. Our changing scope of practice and emerging roles (along with the subsequent need to become more familiar with curricular demands and other academic issues) are discussed in detail. A section of the book is devoted to helping SLPs provide a rationale to the other team members for why we are uniquely suited to address not only speaking

and listening deficits (our traditional milieu) but also reading and writing, which are all language-based processes.

I believe the fact that this book is being written by a practicing SLP with extensive experience in the public school setting (albeit one who is also an academician-researcher) will make the book more appealing to other practicing SLPs and individuals from related disciplines. Unfortunately, because of the perceived gap between research and practice (reinforced by the fact that university faculty and researchers are often no longer involved in "field work" in the public schools), educators and SLPs increasingly tend to believe that research is not relevant to their needs and the needs of their LLD students. I hope to do my part to dispel that myth. I have purposely chosen to remain involved in field work (as a clinical supervisor and clinical service provider working with LLD children and school personnel on a regular basis). By doing so, it is my hope that my work will remain practical, relevant, and useful to SLPs, teachers, and related personnel outside the university setting. Indeed, it is because I wear multiple hats (teacher, researcher, supervisor, clinician) that I feel an even greater responsibility to do my part to bridge the gap between research and practice and to make every effort to unite theory with intervention in language arts.

During preparation of this manuscript, it was decided that a CD-ROM would be made available to accompany the text. The CD-ROM contains the lesson plans, forms for assessment and treatment planning, IEP objectives, protocols for documenting student progress, letters to parents and administrators, sample reports, and other useful handouts that are discussed in detail throughout the text. It is expected that SLPs and related practitioners will want to download and utilize these forms as part of their intervention in language arts on a regular basis.

Acknowledgments

The author would like to extend sincere thanks to the students, teachers, parents, and administrators of Miller Wall Elementary School and Pittman Elementary School, as well as Carolyn Zeller, Betsy Daly, Brandi Townsend, and all the speech-language pathologists in the Jefferson Parish Public School system of Louisiana. Without the students and my outstanding colleagues in Jefferson Parish, this project (and indeed my career) would not have been possible. Special appreciation is also extended to Janet Norris, Ph.D., and Paul Hoffman, Ph.D., at Louisiana State University, Baton Rouge, for providing the author with an outstanding education and many years of mentoring and encouragement. The author would also like to thank her spouse, Ken Ichikawa, and her parents, Maurice and Jeanie DeKemel, for their ongoing encouragement and support. Special recognition and thanks is also extended to my editors, Kellie White, Jennifer Watrous, Doug Turner, and Amanda Carrico, for their expertise and assistance during the completion of this project, as well as to Ms. Jimmie Lyn Harris, Research Librarian at the Texas Woman's University Blagg-Huey Library. Finally, the author would like to express appreciation to Dr. Geraldine Wallach, Clinic Director at California State University, Long Beach, Department of Communication Disorders, for her contributions and considerable body of work in the field of speech-language pathology (work that has greatly influenced this author's evolving understanding of language development and disorders over the years) and for taking the time to review this text and offer her in-depth and insightful commentary in the Foreword.

Biography

Kathryn DeKemel, Ph.D., CCC-SLP is a licensed, certified speech-language pathologist with over 17 years of experience practicing in a variety of settings including public schools, Head Start, private practice, nursing homes, home health, and university clinics. She has extensive experience teaching graduate and undergraduate courses in child language acquisition and language disorders along with other courses in speech-language pathology, as well as a background in clinical supervision and clinical administration. Her research focuses on treatment efficacy studies with school-age language-learning disabled students, the study of narratives and inferential processing, pragmatics (particularly classroom discourse), and exploring the relationship between language and fluency in school-age stutterers.

Contents

Chapter 1
Memory, Inferences, and the Comprehension of Narrative Discourse

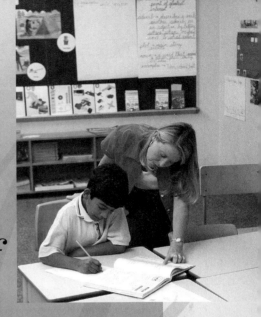

Purposes

- Define the narrative genre.
- Discuss why narratives have become such a popular diagnostic and therapeutic tool for speech-language pathologists and other related professionals.
- Describe the cognitive substrates of narrative comprehension and production.
- Describe the normal developmental sequence of narratives.
- Explore the role of memory and inferential processing in the comprehension of narratives.
- Examine the literature documenting weaknesses in narrative and inferencing abilities in children with specific language and language-learning disabilities.
- Review neuroimaging data pertaining to developmental language disorders and how these data fit with a connectionist-constructionist perspective of narrative discourse comprehension.

Narrative Discourse and Narrative Development

Researchers in a variety of fields including psychology, psycholinguistics, special education, and speech-language pathology have become increasingly interested in **narratives** (Kaderavek and Sulzby, 2000; Schneider, 1996). Narratives (which may be communicated in either the oral or the written modality) mode are essentially stories in which the speaker or writer attempts to communicate some experience not directly shared by the listener or reader. Examples of the narrative genre include telling self-generated stories; telling or retelling familiar stories, folk tales, or fairy tales; recounting the plot of movies or television shows; and recounting personal experiences (Owens, 1991).

Narratives present an attractive medium of study for the following reasons: (1) they provide samples of language in use rather than in isolation, out of context; (2) they comprise a form of language commonly encountered in everyday life, both in social interaction and in recreational and educational media; and (3) they are produced and understood according to certain structural and organizational principles (Schneider, 1996). For these reasons, **speech-language pathologists** (SLPs) and other language practitioners are increasingly using narratives not only as a tool for assessment but as a medium and target for oral and written language intervention, particularly with students who exhibit reading, language, and learning disabilities (Botting, 2002; Greenhalgh & Strong, 2001; Hoggan & Strong, 1994; Kaderavek & Sulzby, 2000; Liles, 1985, 1987, 1993; Merritt & Liles, 1987, 1989; Norris & Hoffman, 1993; Schneider, 1996; Scott & Windsor, 2000).

Research documenting the link between memory, knowledge structures, and narratives has been available for some time. In a review on child memory development published in 1975, Brown reported that children appear to remember best the material that is meaningful to them. In particular, children retain information conveyed in narrative form better than information conveyed in the form of isolated lists. Brown speculated that narratives are more easily remembered are "made to fit the head of the child"; that is, they exist in a format that is already meaningful and familiar. This familiarity exists because narratives are a linguistic universal of sorts, playing a major role in the interpersonal communication of nearly all societies, and because they are produced in some form by people of all ages, with the exception of children younger than 2 years.

Narratives play a major role in our communicative interactions because they have such close correspondence to our daily experiences in contextually specific situations (Bruner, 1986; Kintsch, 1980; Nelson, 1986). In other words, because we know a great deal about people's motives, actions, goals, and attempts to solve daily problems (since it is adaptive to know this information in our social and physical environment), we also come to know a great deal about narratives (Graesser, Singer, & Trabasso, 1994).

In addition to being universally present, narratives also share universality of structure. The consistent, structural components of narratives have been variously referred to as **story grammars** or **story schemata** (Mandler and Johnson, 1977; Rumelhart, 1975; Stein and Glenn, 1979; Thorndyke, 1977). Story grammars typically include elements such as *characters, settings, problems, initiating events, internal responses, plans, attempts, consequences*, and *resolutions*. These elements are important because speakers and writers know (from their experience as communicators in the real world) that they are expected to adhere (more or less) to story grammar structure when communicating narrative information. Readers and listeners also know that they can expect to receive information containing these essential elements. It is the consistency of story grammars, therefore, that ensures that the narrative content will be predictable to communicative participants to a large extent. This predictability is particularly helpful to the reader or listener, whose job in processing and retaining the information is somewhat simplified as a result. Since the reader or listener already has an existing frame or schemata for the narrative, the information conveyed is generally much easier to process, store, and retrieve in comparison to information conveyed in other more isolated formats.

Note that because most theoretical claims in this book apply equally to language and participants across the modalities—that is, speakers, listeners, readers, and writers—I have dispensed with the awkward *listener/reader* and *speaker/writer* designations, with the understanding that claims refer to communicative modalities and communicative participants in general, regardless of whether the communication takes place in the spoken or written mode. Also, I have decided to dispense with the endless and awkward arguments concerning the definitions of terms such as *language-learning disabled* (LLD) and *Specific Language Impairment* (SLI) when referring to the population of children with whom we are concerned throughout this book. Let us agree that I will use these terms fairly interchangeably to refer to the population of students we serve in the schools who exhibit "spoken language disorders, written language disorders, receptive and expressive language disorders, spoken *and* written language disorders, language-based reading and writing deficits, language delays, language impairments," and the like. It is generally understood and accepted that these children exhibit such language difficulties in the absence of overt sensory impairments and that they have intelligence in the "normal" range.

Development of Narratives in Children

Various authors (Applebee, 1978; Liles, 1993; Owens, 1991) have investigated narrative development in children, and discernible patterns of acquisition have emerged (Box 1-1). Although it is generally agreed that most children are capable of producing an ideal, adult-type narrative by 6 to 7 years of age, narrative form and content continue to be refined throughout late childhood and adolescence (Liles, 1993). This later development is often characterized by an increased number of episodes in the narrative, as well as an increased ability to link multiple episodes together in complex ways (Purcell & Liles, 1992; Roth & Spekman, 1986).

Box 1-1 Developmental Sequence for Narratives

Ages 2 to 3 Years

Prenarratives; additive chains; heaps; descriptive or action sequences

Children talk about whatever attracts their attention, but without specifying relationships among the elements; characters, objects, and events are put together because they are perceptually associated with each other; there is no macrostructure; there is no real plot or story line; there is no discernible beginning, middle, or end, and no specific order of events; there are no cause-effect relationships.

Ages 3 to 5 Years

Primitive narratives; temporal event sequences; causal chains

There is still no well-developed theme or plot, but characters, objects, and events are put together because they complement each other in some logical way; events are linked sequentially or causally; there may be a beginning and middle but no ending or resolution.

Ages 6 to 7 Years

True narratives

Narratives contain a fully developed plot and a clear beginning, middle, and ending; logical cause-effect relationships are specified and linked to the macrostructure of the story; there is increased character development; narratives contain markers such as *once upon a time, lived happily ever after, the end*; narratives contain dialogue and may contain evaluative statements such as *"That was a good one."*

Ages 8 and Older

Complex narratives

Narratives have continued plot development; stories increase in length and complexity with embedding of multiple episodes; there is increased use of syntactic devices such as conjunctions (*and, then*), locatives (*in, on, under, next to*), comparatives (*almost, bigger than*), and adjectives; there are fewer unresolved problems and more resolutions; there are fewer extraneous details; narratives have a better introduction, including a setting; there is more overt marking of changes in time and place as well as better description of characters' motives and internal responses; narratives show a closer adherence to a story grammar model.

Modified from The Child's Concept of Story, *by A. Applebee, 1978, Chicago: University of Chicago Press and "Narrative Analysis," by R. Owens, in* Language Disorders: A Functional Approach to Assessment and Intervention, *1991, Columbus, OH: Macmillan.*

Inferencing and Narrative Comprehension

An ability that is intrinsically linked with the comprehension of narratives is that of **inferencing**. Brown and Yule (1983) define inferencing as "that process which the hearer or reader must go through to get from the literal meaning of what is said/written to what the speaker/writer intended to convey." In other words, listeners and readers cannot rely exclusively on explicitly stated information to achieve comprehension. They must go beyond what is explicitly or literally stated in the text to grasp subtleties and implied nuances of meaning. This is not to say, however, that text-based information is unimportant. Rather, to draw plausible,

appropriate inferences, the communicator must combine prior knowledge with text-based information in order to accurately reconstruct the intended meaning (Anderson, Reynolds, Schallert, & Goetz, 1977; Anderson, Spiro, & Anderson, 1978; Bishop & Adams, 1992; McCormick, 1992).

To illustrate how the inferencing phenomenon works, consider the following brief examples from Nicholas and Trabasso (1980):

1. *Mary had a little lamb. Its fleece was white as snow.*
2. *Mary had a little lamb. She spilled gravy and mint jelly on her dress.*
3. *Mary had a little lamb. The delivery was difficult and afterwards the vet needed a drink.*

In item 1, the reader will probably infer that Mary is the little girl from a well-known nursery rhyme who is followed by her pet lamb. In item 2, the reader will likely infer that Mary is dining on lamb, either at home or perhaps at a restaurant. The reader may further infer that Mary is a little girl (since children often spill food on themselves) or, conversely, that Mary is a very old woman (as elderly people may also have difficulty eating and swallowing, due to loss of muscle control, dentures, and other factors) or that Mary (regardless of age) is simply a messy eater. Alternately, the reader may infer nothing at all about Mary's age, traits, or personality from these two statements, preferring to wait for additional text-based information before drawing any conclusions. In item 3, the reader will likely infer that Mary is not human at all, but rather a mature female sheep who has just given birth to a lamb, and that the veterinarian who presided at the birth needed a drink to relax after the hard work involved in the delivery.

These examples illustrate that a considerable amount of world or background knowledge is needed in order to make inferences about information not explicitly stated in the text. For instance, to make sense of the text, the reader of the previous passages would need to possess and activate prior knowledge structures associated with a variety of topics, including familiar nursery rhymes, owning a pet, characteristics and traits of little girls and old women, dining at home or in a restaurant, caring for farm animals, veterinarians, animal births, and alcoholic beverages (Trabasso & Nicholas, 1980). However, although activation of relevant background knowledge is clearly an important factor, it is also necessary to achieve a best-fit solution that preserves the cohesive relationship and propositional ties between the two sentences in each passage. Text-based, explicit information is clearly important as well, and plausible inferences cannot be generated unless the relationships specified in the literal text are preserved during the reconstruction of meaning by the reader.

Inferencing as Constructive Comprehension

Many theoretical frameworks have been used to define and explain inferencing behavior in relation to discourse processing. As previously stated, read-

ers do not achieve comprehension simply by decoding the literal meaning of the text (Bishop & Adams, 1992). The reader must also utilize contextual information and stored background knowledge to fill in the gaps or infer what has not been explicitly stated. This process of filling in the gaps has been variously referred to as *constructive comprehension* (Westby, 1984), *goodness of fit analysis* (Wallach & Miller, 1988), *developing an inferential set* (Hansen & Pearson, 1983), and *search (or effort) after meaning* (Bartlett, 1932; Berlyne, 1949, 1960; Graesser et al., 1994; Spiro, 1980; Stein and Trabasso, 1985). The ability to engage in constructive comprehension is critical, for, as noted by Weaver and Kintsch (1983), "[t]here can be as many as 12 to 15 implicit inferences for every expressly mentioned statement" in a passage of narrative or expository text. Samuels and Kamil (1984) also note that "even the simplest type of literal comprehension requires that we engage in inferencing." Taken together, these findings suggest that the reader must continually make inferences in order to comprehend even the smallest pieces of text. Considering the integral part inferencing plays in text comprehension, it is not surprising that researchers such as Winne, Graham, and Prock (1993) have referred to this ability as "a cornerstone of reading competence."

Development of Inferencing Abilities in Children

As with narrative development, studies show that inferencing abilities in children also develop in predictable ways, and that by the age of 6 to 7 years, most children are fairly skilled at making adult-type inferences. However, as with narrative development, some aspects of inferential processing appear to continue to develop through the middle grades (Wallach & Miller, 1988). The apparent similarity in the ages at which children are simultaneously capable of producing fully developed narratives and making adult-type inferences may be related to their reaching certain cognitive developmental milestones. The time frame in question (ages 6 to 7 years) coincides with the child's transition from the *preoperational stage* to the *concrete operations stage* (Piaget, 1952, 1954, 1960). During the preoperational stage (ages 2 to 7 years), children rely almost exclusively on the immediate perceptual characteristics of objects to construct a framework of reality, and they trust as valid only what they perceive. Therefore, although children at this stage may be capable of describing a simple series of actions or events (based on perception), they are often incapable of describing logical cause-effect relationships between actions and events, or attributing complex motives to characters in a story (both of which are largely dependent on inferencing, because authors frequently do not specify these relationships explicitly in the story). On entering the concrete operations stage (ages 7 through 11 or 12 years), the child's thinking is no longer dominated by simple perception, and operations such as classification, seriation, coordination, reversibility, and conservation are acquired. These new operations allow the child to understand more advanced concepts of temporality and causality in narratives, as well as changes in state.

The continued development in narrative and inferencing abilities that occurs in late childhood or adolescence may be related to the child's transition from concrete operations to the *formal operations stage* (ages 11 or 12 through 14 or 15 years). On reaching the formal operations stage, the child is finally able to perform purely mental operations on nonconcrete objects, exhibit complete generality of thought, engage in propositional thinking, and deal with hypothetical situations and events. This move toward the formal operations stage may be reflected in the child's increased ability to attribute complex motives to characters; understand abstract relationships between problems, plans, attempts, and solutions; and predict possible consequences or outcomes of events in a story. In other words, as children's cognitive abilities become increasingly more elaborated over time, their narratives become increasingly more elaborated as well, and they also become more adept at making inferences about the kind of information that is often not explicitly stated in the narrative text.

Theoretical Models of Inferencing

Given the interest in exploring the link between memory, inferences, and the comprehension of narratives, considerable debate has arisen about the extent to which inferencing and comprehension are **text-based** or **schema-based** phenomena (Carnine, Kameenui, & Woolfson, 1982). Proponents of text-based theory have traditionally analyzed textual characteristics such as thematic organization, sentence structure, propositional structure, and cohesion, whereas advocates of schema-based models have emphasized the role of the reader's prior knowledge structures (including story schema knowledge and general world knowledge) in comprehension (Carnine et al., 1982). Other theorists have proposed a balance between the two paradigms by asserting that it is the reader's ability to blend knowledge of textual characteristics with prior knowledge that accounts for "correct" or plausible inferencing. Hansen (1981), for example, suggests that when information is not explicitly stated in the text, a reciprocal process takes place, whereby the reader uses textual information to instantiate a probable schema, then makes a guess, or inference, according to what would best fit that schema. The reader then checks the inference against additional incoming textual information, activates a different or modified schema as needed, makes a new or adjusted inference, rechecks the text, and so on, until a best fit between prior knowledge structures and textual information is achieved. Hansen describes this process as making **default assignments** and indicates that a reader who relies too heavily on either text-based information or prior knowledge risks making incorrect or faulty inferences. According to Hansen's model, it is the reader's ability to balance and blend text-based information with prior knowledge to achieve best-fit solutions that results in the generation of plausible or correct inferences and maximal reconstruction of intended meaning.

Researchers have proposed several taxonomies to describe the different types of inferences that are generated during the comprehension of narrative text. Several of these taxonomies are based on the premise that comprehension consists of the construction of multilevel representations of texts, and that comprehension improves to the extent that the reader constructs more levels of representation and more inferences at each level (Graesser et al., 1994). For instance, under the overall category of **knowledge-based inferences,** Graesser et al. differentiate between *shallow* low-level inferences that are instantiated to construct propositional code, syntactic code, and the explicit textbase, and *deeper* high-level inferences, which involve the reader's inferring the global message or point of the text (including causes and motives that explain why actions or events have occurred). According to their definition of comprehension, Graesser et al. indicate that it is the reader's job to construct representations of meaning at both shallow and deep levels. To illustrate these phenomena, they propose the following example:

> *The truck driver saw the policeman hold up his hand. The truck driver's vehicle stopped, but a car rear-ended the truck driver.*

An analysis of the textbase or shallow level of representation in this passage (Kintsch, 1992; Kintsch & Van Dijk, 1978) reveals the following propositional content of the first sentence:

Proposition 1: saw (truck driver, proposition 2)
Proposition 2: hold up (policeman, hand)

At the textbase level, each of these propositions has a predicate (i.e., verb, connective, or adjective) and one or more arguments (i.e., noun or embedded proposition), and the two sentences are connected by the overlapping argument *truck driver*. But this shallow level of representation still fails to capture the deeper, more global meaning of the text. Deeper comprehension can only be achieved when the reader infers causes and motives to explain why the events occurred. For example, a reader would likely infer the following: (1) the policeman held up his hand with the goal of having the truck driver stop his vehicle (perhaps for safety reasons or to control the flow of traffic); (2) it was an abrupt stop on the part of the truck driver (in response to the policeman's holding up his hand to indicate "Stop!") that triggered the accident, when the car behind the truck could not stop in time to avoid a collision; and (3) the car rear-ended the vehicle of the truck driver and not the truck driver himself, as the explicit text would seem to suggest. The reader would also infer that the truck driver performed some action to stop the truck (such as stepping on the brake), as did the driver of the car (although the action was unsuccessful in preventing the collision), and that the truck driver had the goal of stopping in order to avoid getting a ticket from the policeman (or because drivers are expected to respond to a policeman's directions in traffic for safety reasons). The driver of the car also had the goal of stopping in an attempt to avoid hitting the truck. Finally, the reader might make a more global inference about the passage, such as "Accidents occur even when people follow the rules," or "It is dangerous to follow too closely behind another vehicle in traffic." It is readily apparent that the inferences generated while attempting to construct meaning from this passage rely quite heavily on prior knowledge and experience, and that the number of inferences that may or must be drawn to construct the various levels of meaning are almost endless. Obviously, the more inferences the reader constructs (both shallow and deep), the richer and more multilayered the comprehension of the text.

Graesser et al. (1994) advocate a **constructionist theory** of comprehension to explain the mechanism by which readers generate inferences during the actual reading of the text, as opposed to generating inferences during some later retrieval task. According to Graesser et al., "all knowledge-based inferences generated while reading the text are constructed when background knowledge structures in **long-term memory** are activated." Background knowledge consists of both generic knowledge structures (i.e., meaningful, contextually rich packets of knowledge such as scripts or schemata), as well as specific knowledge structures that are relevant to the text (including memory representations of other texts, and of prior excerpts within the same text). Graesser et al. propose that background knowledge structures are first activated through pattern recognition by explicit content words, combinations of content words, or interpreted text constituents. When knowledge structures from long-term memory are activated, a subset of this information is then encoded in the meaning representation of the text, which includes both the textbase and a referential situation model (i.e., a mental representation of the setting, characters, actions, and events that are mentioned explicitly or that are filled-in inferentially from world or background knowledge). Graesser and Clark (1985) and Kintsch (1988) further suggest that when a background knowledge structure is very familiar, much of the content for that memory structure is automatically activated in **working memory**, at a very small cost to the processing resources. In other words, according to constructionist theory, when a knowledge-based inference is "directly inherited" or copied from a background knowledge structure (due to high familiarity), the process of incorporating it into the meaning representation of the text places very little processing burden on the reader's working memory. On the other hand, sometimes a novel knowledge-based inference must be constructed. Such a novel inference might involve several cycles of searching memory for the appropriate background knowledge structures to make the inference (Graesser et al., 1994; Just and Carpenter, 1992). Theoretically, generation of these novel inferences would place a much higher burden on working memory; thus, a potential inference has less likelihood of being generated to the extent that it imposes higher demands on working memory.

Connectionist Models and Solving the Frame Problem

Although constructionist theory is appealing in many ways (particularly as it specifies how inferences may actually be generated), it fails to solve what has been referred to as the **frame problem.** The frame problem may be summarized as follows: When polymodal input is being received from the environment (for example, when humans are trying to read and process narrative text), theoretically, any part of the **total knowledge base** of the individual may be relevant for making the necessary inferences at any given point in time. Garfield (1990) notes that the frame problem, or "the problem of how we organize knowledge and information about the world in such a way that the relevant bits are available when they are needed, without having to perform an exhaustive or horrendously inefficient search of the listener's knowledge base," has yet to be satisfactorily resolved in the field of cognitive science. Interestingly, the frame problem also continues to pose a major stumbling block in the field of artificial intelligence. Put simply, solving the frame problem remains staggeringly difficult for current artificial intelligence machines but appears to pose little difficulty for normally intelligent humans (Garfield, 1990). In fact, inference generation (along with question asking and answering, summary generation, and paraphrasing) has traditionally served as a sort of litmus test of whether artificial intelligence computers are capable of understanding text (Graesser et al., 1994; Kass, 1992; Lehnert, Dyer, Johnson, Yang & Harley, 1983; Schank & Abelson, 1977). Further exploration of how (and by what mechanism) relevant background information is stored and activated efficiently, easily, and at the right time by humans may shed light on how to facilitate this

process in the next generation of artificial intelligence computers.

In summary, we know that humans process narrative discourse quite rapidly, yet it would be almost impossible to engage in the kind of rapid processing needed to make sense of the text if we had to filter through our entire store of background knowledge to determine which information is relevant every time we needed to make an inference. To make inferences, we require the ability (and indeed appear to have the ability) to determine which previous background knowledge structures are relevant and to activate the pattern associated with that knowledge almost instantaneously. In addition we must also determine which information from the continuing stream of input data (i.e., the continuing textbase of the narrative) is relevant, so that we can confirm or deny the schemata initially activated, and/or modify the inference accordingly.

Although constructionist theory does specify that background information that is highly familiar somehow places less demand on working memory, the exact mechanism for how information might actually be stored or accessed in working memory or long-term memory is unspecified. Perhaps before attempting to design a model for how the system solves the frame problem, it is necessary to reexamine the larger question of how humans acquire and store knowledge (particularly knowledge about routine events and story structure) and how they retrieve or activate this knowledge. A **connectionist** or **parallel distributed processing** (PDP) model of cognition (grafted onto the existing framework of the constructionist model) may do a better job of explaining how individuals store and access knowledge of routine events and story structure, as well as how they solve the frame problem in order to generate inferences quickly and accurately.

Generalized Event Representations

First let us examine how children's knowledge of routine events is acquired. According to Nelson (1985; 1986; 1991), **scripts,** or "**generalized event representations,**" describe children's schematic knowledge of routine events. It is through the child's active participation in routine events (e.g., eating, bathing, napping, dressing, going to the store, or reading a storybook) that these event representations are created. Initially, the child perceives the event holistically and does not separate the parts (i.e., people, actions, objects, outcomes) from the whole. But as the caregiver talks to the child and points out the salient aspects of these routine events, the child becomes aware of the elements involved and gradually builds a network of associations representing the entire event. These representations include specification of the event's temporal and causal structure, its obligatory and optional components, and the props and roles commonly associated with the event. Young children's basic event knowledge is thought to be very similar to that of an adult's in terms of both its schematic structure and its consistency across time and individuals. Event representations constitute one of the child's earliest and most stable forms of knowledge about the world and form the basic building blocks for subsequent cognitive development.

PDP models of cognition attempt to show how such conceptual information may be represented in neural networks, where connections between bits of information (units) are activated as a pattern across the network, representing a concept or event. The connections between units, or **connection weights,** have variable strengths that undergo continuous adjustment based on experience. Events or routines that the child encounters frequently in life result in stronger connection weights between the units representing the concept or event. Theoretically, stronger connection weights would result in easier access and retrieval of the concept as well. For instance, in the Nicholas and Trabasso (1980) "Mary had a little lamb" example previously cited, hearing and singing the familiar nursery rhyme over and over (as many children do) would result in strong connection weights for the pattern of activation representing that event or concept. Newer or less frequently encountered events (e.g., eating lamb, or watching a sheep give birth) would have much weaker connection weights between units. PDP models stipulate that anything that has been previously learned or experienced may be reactivated within the network at any time (for example, when the reader encountered the first "Mary had a little lamb" sample sentence earlier in this chapter). The pattern that is initially activated by this incoming data is the one with the strongest connection weights (for most of us, certainly, the familiar nursery rhyme event representation). Therefore, this highly familiar pattern is activated immediately, before we even read or process the

second sentence in the passage (similar to the phenomena Hansen referred to as making default assignments). We activate patterns with weaker connection weights only when subsequent stimuli (in this case the text-based data concerning gravy and mint jelly) force us to reject the first, more likely, representation. In other words, rather than focusing on an artificial dichotomy between working memory and long-term memory and suggesting that there are fewer processing demands when information is overlearned, the emphasis in PDP models is on concepts consisting of patterns of activation of units across a network, with stronger connection weights between units resulting from experience leading to easier access and retrieval of that concept.

Finding a Best-Fit Solution: A Constructionist-Connectionist Model of Inferencing

Although PDP models go a long way toward solving the frame dilemma, one more component remains to be added. A **constructionist-connectionist** model that would allow the reader to make use of simultaneous bottom-up and top-down processing in order to construct a best-fit solution to the inference may solve the frame problem, since it would never be necessary to activate the entire store of prior knowledge all at once. Such a model would work as follows. Initial input to the system (primarily from the textbase) activates the most likely schemata or representation (i.e., bottom-up processing) because the connection weights for this pattern of activation are stronger owing to experience. Therefore the **first-guess inference,** or default solution, is generated quickly and easily and has a high probability of being correct. However, the system also has a "safeguard" mechanism in the form of almost simultaneous top-down processing in order to handle contradictions that may arise from subsequent incoming data. While instantiating the first schema and inference, the system quickly scans the continuously incoming data stream to confirm or deny the plausibility of the inference. If a match or best-fit solution is achieved, the default inference is retained. However, if subsequent data from the input stream deny the plausibility of the first-guess inference, we must resort to activating the patterns for a series of less likely schemata and formulating new or modified inferences, which are tested against incoming data, and so forth, until a best-fit solution is achieved. In this manner, the system is designed for speed and maximal efficiency in activating appropriate background knowledge (without having to search the entire knowledge store) but is also equipped with safeguards that allow flexibility in generating alternate solutions as needed, through simultaneous top-down and bottom-up processing.

Some preliminary neurophysiological evidence suggests that the brain is capable of and does engage in simultaneous top-down and bottom-up processing. Specifically, reciprocal interactions between the **reticular formation** (RF), cerebellum, hippocampus, and cortex (particularly the prefrontal cortex) may be involved in this process.

The RF has been described as a *universal connector* or *gating mechanism* for all the parts of the brain (Parkins, 1990). In addition to connecting the cerebellum and the cerebrum to the environment, the RF may also facilitate interaction between the cerebellum and the cerebrum. It is now known that the cerebellum has fiber tracts that connect it directly with all major subdivisions of the cerebral cortex and that it may influence electrical activity in all four lobes of the brain, including cerebral responses to external stimuli. Additionally, evidence suggests that the cerebellum may activate or influence neurons within the RF, possibly exerting some sort of discriminatory control. Through the ascending RF, the cortex appears to receive nonspecific, polymodal input, the content of which is thought to be experientially based and related to the contextual significance of the stimuli. This may provide the equivalent of a *psychological set* (similar to an inferential set) that serves as background for subsequent cerebrocortical processing (Parkins, 1990). This process may be twofold. First, the data concerning the contextual significance of the stimuli may be forwarded to the cortex through the ascending RF. Second, on the basis of this information, the cortex may selectively attend to or filter subsequent ascending information by means of its influence on the reticular system through cerebroreticular projections (Parkins, 1990).

The hippocampus also appears to be significantly involved with attention, memory, and the activation of relevant background knowledge. Although it is not the site of actual memory storage, the hippocampus appears to act as a key of access to the experiential record, or memory bank (Parkins, 1990). Specifically, the hippocampus seems to be involved in the mechanism that allows information to be consciously retrieved from the memory bank (where all our previous experiences are recorded), and it also influences input to the cerebrum through its reticular connections. Clearly, the cerebellum, the hippocampus, and the RF are involved in a complex reciprocal process whereby information is filtered and directed back and forth between the cerebrum and the environment, and the resulting comparison between incoming stimuli and relevant stored information is involved in memory storage, retrieval, and inferencing.

New findings garnered from neuroimaging studies are also providing support for top-down–bottom-up connectionist-constructionist models of processing and memory. **Positron emission tomography** (PET) is a brain-scanning technique that provides a precise reading of blood flow in localized brain regions (Schacter, 1996). The underlying rationale for PET is that when a region of the brain is actively involved in a specific cognitive task, that area should become more active, thus requiring more blood uptake (Schacter, 1996). Another neuroimaging technique called **functional magnetic resonance imaging** (functional MRI or fMRI) also measures changes in regional blood flow during the performance of cognitive tasks. Researchers have been successful in using PET and fMRI to explore activation patterns and blood flow during a variety of memory storage, retrieval, and other cognitive tasks. For instance, Kapur, Craik, Jones, Brown, Houle, and Tulving (1995) found evidence that there is strong activation (i.e., high blood flow) in the left inferior prefrontal cortex associated with **elaborative encoding** (i.e., the process by which subjects make a conscious effort to remember by associating new information with previous knowledge). These results have been confirmed using fMRI (Schacter, 1996). Likewise, the hippocampus, which has previously been implicated as a structure important for memory access and retrieval, also appears to be involved during elaborative encoding (Schacter, 1996). Neuroimaging results suggest that part of the encoding process (i.e., the process of transforming something a human thinks, feels, hears, or sees into a memory) involves a hippocampal response to novelty. When the hippocampus becomes active during exposure to a novel event, the individual's attention is drawn to the event. Furthermore, there appears to be a reciprocal relationship between activation of the hippocampus in response to novelty and activation of other areas of the brain presumed to store relevant memories and prior knowledge. Schacter (1996) reported PET results that suggest that once the hippocampus is activated by a novel stimulus, another network presumed to store a wealth of semantic associations and prior knowledge (specifically a region of the left inferior frontal lobe) is then activated as well. According to Schacter, it is this interaction between the hippocampus and the left inferior frontal lobe that allows us to engage in elaborative encoding (i.e., the process of integrating new information with existing knowledge), and elaborative encoding in turn yields a higher probability that the new information will be readily recalled or retrieved at a later time.

Along similar lines, Moscovitch (1994) has suggested that the frontal and hippocampal systems may actually be involved in two different types of memory retrieval. Moscovitch uses the term **associative retrieval** to refer to the process whereby a retrieval cue automatically triggers an experience of remembering (for example, when hearing an old song inadvertently triggers a memory of where you were, whom you were with, and what you were doing when you used to hear that song). Moscovitch suggests that associative retrieval probably depends on the hippocampus and other related medial temporal lobe structures. On the other hand, Moscovitch proposes that **effortful retrieval,** or **strategic retrieval** (i.e., the process whereby we explicitly and effortfully try to retrieve prior knowledge or memories), most likely involves activation of regions of the prefrontal cortex (as indicated in PET studies).

Although still preliminary, results from these neuroimaging studies lend credence to the notion that *there is no single location or area in the brain that contains the memory of a particular experience or event*, and that *different brain regions work reciprocally and collaboratively during the processes of encoding, filtering, and retrieving stored information*. This notion is hardly new; memory researchers as far back as Semon (1904/1921, 1909/1923) have been interested in what constitutes the **engram**, or actual neural representation of a memory in the brain. Semon argued that memory consists of **engraphy** (his term for the process of encoding information into memory), the engram

itself (the enduring change in the nervous system, or memory trace), and **ecphory** (the process of activating and retrieving a memory). What made Semon's work so different from that of his contemporaries was that he focused not only on the process of memory storage (a popular subject for exploration and discussion at the time) but also on memory retrieval. Many neuroscientists believed then (as many continue to believe now) that the likelihood of remembering an experience or event is determined by the strength of connections or associations formed when that event was initially encoded into memory. Semon further argued, however, that memory does not solely depend on the strength of the associations or connections made at the time of encoding. Rather he suggested that the probability of remembering also depends strongly on the hints or cues that trigger recall (he called these hints or cues the **ecphoric stimulus**) and how the cues are related to the original engram or memory trace.

Although his work was largely ignored at the time, some of Semon's ideas did become an enduring part of the neuroscience literature (particularly his notion of the engram), and other neuroscientists have continued to suggest that the brain stores an engram by strengthening connections between groups of neurons that participated in the encoding experience. This theory closely parallels modern connectionist–neural network theories of brain organization. As Schacter (1996) notes, any typical experience from our lives generally consists of multimodal input (i.e., sights, sounds, smells, tactile sensations, feelings, etc.). Different areas of the brain (e.g., regions of the parietal, occipital, and temporal lobes) appear to be responsible for analyzing various aspects of this input in order to make sense of the whole event. As a result, neurons in different regions of the brain eventually become more strongly connected to one another as a result of experience. The particular pattern of these connections constitutes the brain's record of the event or the engram (Hebb, 1949; Schacter, 1996). Engrams are thus important contributors to the subjective experience of remembering and using stored information for performing various cognitive tasks (such as inferencing). Presumably, at any given moment, there may be millions of engrams existing in the brain in the form of patterns of neural connections. These patterns have the potential to enter our awareness and contribute to implicit, associative, unintentional recall, or to explicit, effortful, intentional recall at any given time. An external retrieval cue from the environment, or an internal retrieval cue (both of which may well exist as a unit or piece of the original engram), may activate the entire engram or pattern of connections at a particular time. But most patterns simply lie dormant or inactivated until they are needed. The strength of this theory (and a strength of connectionist theories in general) is that only a fraction of the original event or a tiny piece of the engram in the form of an internal or external cue needs to be present to trigger activation and recall of the entire episode or event. Once again this helps to solve the frame problem by explaining how we are able to activate relevant prior knowledge (i.e., a particular engram) when needed without having to engage in an exhaustive search of our entire memory bank. More importantly, connectionist theory helps us to view both memory storage and retrieval as dynamic, fluid, reciprocal processes, with memory in general existing as a constructed, transitional entity or work in progress, consisting of a constantly changing network of associations strengthened through experience and repeated activation. Connectionism can also help us explain the phenomenon of forgetting, or failing to retrieve relevant stored information at the appropriate time. Engrams whose connections are not strengthened through experience and repeated activation are more likely to fade gradually over time and thus may be more difficult to activate when needed. Most importantly, connectionist models encourage us not to ignore the importance of retrieval cues on the memory process. Some proponents such as Schacter (1996) go even further by suggesting that a memory is not merely an activated engram but a uniquely new activation pattern that emerges from the pooled contributions of the retrieval cue and the stored engram. In this light, there is no need for false dichotomies to exist between phenomena such as memory storage, retrieval, and the coalescing of new information with prior knowledge. Instead, all these processes operate in parallel as part of a flexible, emergent, collaborative neural network that is capable of handling a variety of complex cognitive tasks (including inferencing) effectively and efficiently.

What does all this talk of engrams and memory and neuroimaging have to do with children who exhibit language and learning disabilities? As we will see in the following sections, evidence is emerging that LLD children's inability to make plausible inferences is one critical source of their narrative and reading comprehension difficulties (and thus it is a problem that spreads across the language arts curriculum). Indeed, the intertwined nature of their difficulties with memory, inferences, and the comprehension of narratives (and how to treat those deficits) forms the basis of much of the remainder of this text.

Language-Learning–Disabled Children's Difficulties With Narratives and Inferencing

Researchers have documented a variety of weaknesses in the narratives of LLD children. In general, their narratives are shorter and less complex than those produced by their age-matched peers, with deficits apparent in overall length and complexity, story grammar constituents, sentence grammar, content, and cohesion (Gillam, 1989; Gillam & Johnston, 1992; Graybeal, 1981; Liles, 1985, 1987, 1993; Merritt & Liles, 1987). Recent research is providing even more documentation of narrative deficits in this population, across different genres in the oral and written modalities (Greenhalgh & Strong, 2001; Kaderavek & Sulzby, 2000; Scott & Windsor, 2000; Wright & Newhoff, 2001). LLD children's inferencing problems, in conjunction with their more global narrative deficits, have the potential to negatively affect their performance in a variety of academic areas. It is not surprising that these children find themselves unable to adequately comprehend and explain story actions, events, and character motives; answer comprehension questions about stories; explain cause-effect relationships; and otherwise summarize or retell narrative information in correct sequence and detail. All of the above abilities would be expected of children at least by third or fourth grade, as they make the transition in the language arts curriculum from *learning to read* to *reading to learn*.

Although it is accepted that proficient readers and listeners make inferences regularly and with relative ease, studies suggest that even normal children and adults sometimes have difficulty making inferences (Bransford et al., 1982; Davey & Macready, 1985; Holmes, 1985; Paris & Lindauer, 1976; Wilson, 1979; Winne et al., 1993). The literature on inferential processing suggests that both children and adults typically have more difficulty answering inferential questions than factual or literal questions about stories (Holmes, 1985; Pearson et al., 1979). From the 1990s through the early 2000s researchers have focused on exploring the narrative and inferential processing abilities of LLD children, who appear to have greater problems in these areas in comparison with their normal peers.

Several researchers (Bishop & Adams, 1992; Crais & Chapman, 1987; DeKemel, 1998; Ellis-Weismer, 1985; Wong, 1980) have investigated LLD children's ability to process implied information by presenting them with short story sequences or complete stories (presented either by reading the story, showing pictures, or having the subjects read the story aloud) and subsequently having the children answer a series of factual and inference-type questions. The LLD children's performance was then compared with that of same-age (age-matched) normal language peers as well as younger, language-age–, or in some cases, reading-age–matched peers. Results from these studies have yielded fairly consistent results in that the LLD children generally performed more poorly than their normal language-age–matched peers on both types of questions but performed similarly to their younger, language-age–matched and reading-age–matched peers. These findings have led researchers to speculate that *LLD children have the ability to infer but may need specific help in learning how to apply inferential processing strategies*. It has been further suggested that because LLD children do not appear to impose structure on stories and do not engage in constructive comprehension, they are poor at understanding and remembering all aspects of a story, including both implied and explicitly stated information. This hypothesis is consistent with other research findings (Liles, 1993; Norris and Hoffman, 1993) that suggest that SLI-LLD children exhibit difficulty with various global aspects of narrative comprehension and production.

Potential Causes of Inferential Processing Deficits in Language-Learning–Disabled or Poor Readers

A number of other theories have been offered to explain why students in general (and in particular those with reading and language-learning disabili-

ties) sometimes have difficulty answering inference-type questions about stories in particular. One possible reason is a lack of practice with this question type. Hansen and Pearson (1983) note that although children infer naturally and regularly during their nonschool lives (by attempting to infer similarities and differences between new situations and those they have already encountered), they are seldom required to infer during their school lives. Evidence suggests that teachers generally ask more literal than inferential-type questions in the classroom (Guszak, 1967) and that lower-achieving students in particular are asked fewer inferential questions than are better readers (Chou-Hare & Pulliam, 1980; Palmer, 1982; Sadker & Sadker, 1982). In fact, poor readers are more likely to be involved in lessons that emphasize word identification and decoding skills as opposed to comprehension (Winne et al., 1993). Kos (1991) notes that in general, little instructional time is devoted to comprehension in most classrooms, and even less to inferential comprehension (Kos, 1991). Hansen and Pearson (1983) also point out that rather than being taught to learn textual information by relating it to something familiar (thus leading to activation of appropriate schemata), children are often encouraged to learn new information simply by memorizing it. Given the lack of emphasis on comprehension and the resulting lack of inferencing practice, it is not surprising that many school-age readers exhibit inferential processing abilities that are less well developed than those needed for literal comprehension.

Still other theories have focused on the reader's ability (or lack thereof) to activate relevant background knowledge as a potential source of inferencing difficulties. First, readers may simply lack the appropriate background knowledge needed to make the necessary inference (Pearson, Hansen, & Gordon, 1979). Second, they may possess the appropriate prior knowledge but underutilize it for a variety of reasons. Spiro and Myers (1984) suggest that readers may underutilize prior knowledge because (1) they are unable to determine which schemata to draw upon, (2) they lack appropriate strategies for activating and retrieving relevant schemata, (3) they do not maintain activation of the schemata for a sufficient period of time, (4) they have a confused representation of knowledge, or (5) they pay undue attention to word decoding or identification, thus exceeding their

---

Box 1-2   Reasons Why Language-Learning–Disabled Students May Have Difficulty Instantiating Plausible Inferences

- They may focus on irrelevant information from the text, rather than picking up on salient cues that would lead to activation of an appropriate schema for instantiating a plausible inference.
- They may fail to update the default inference as new or contrasting information becomes available from the textbase.
- They may lack appropriate background knowledge for instantiating a plausible inference.
- They may underutilize background knowledge (possibly due to memory retrieval problems, confused representation of knowledge, poor organization of schemata).
- They may spend so much time struggling with word decoding that they exceed their processing capacity.
- Word identification or decoding problems may deny access to salient text-based meaning clues.
- They may overutilize background or prior knowledge (they may have trouble differentiating what has actually been stated in the text from what they perceive has been stated, based on prior knowledge; an inability to fully comprehend the textbase may cause overreliance on prior knowledge).
- They may be unaware of inferencing strategies and the importance of blending text-based information with prior knowledge.
- They may have a lack of practice answering interpretation and inference questions (because of the teacher's preference for factual questions, especially for poor readers).

---

processing capacity limitations. Third, readers may exhibit an overreliance on prior knowledge when making inferences. Anderson (1978) proposed that readers may be unable to differentiate between what has actually been stated in the text and what they perceive to be logical based on prior information, resulting in the generation of inferences too heavily shaded by previous perceptions. Spiro and Myers (1984) also suggest that excessive word identification problems in some readers may limit their access to text-based information, thus inducing them to rely too heavily on background knowledge to make sense of the text. Finally, Tierney and Pearson (1981) note that some readers may simply be unaware of strategies for drawing inferences (specifically, that inferencing requires a coalescence of text information and prior knowledge) and may exhibit a lack of flexibility in using either background information or written, text-based clues for making various inferences. Any of these circumstances may cause the reader to make inferences that Tierney and Pearson describe as being *too text-based* (i.e., based too heavily on literal information from the text) or *too reader-based* (i.e., based too much on the reader's prior knowledge). Box 1-2 contains a summary of why LLD students may have difficulty making plausible inferences.

Much work remains to be done in the area of determining what causes memory, inferencing, and narrative deficits in the LLD population. It is only with a better understanding of *why* these children struggle with processes that appear to come easily and naturally to children who are acquiring language normally that we will be able to design better intervention programs.

Recent Neuroimaging Research on Developmental Language Disorders

Although neuroimaging studies were mentioned earlier in the chapter (the work of Daniel Schacter, specifically), it is important to note that these studies were done on *adults*, not children. Also, although there is a consensus that the brains of individuals with developmental language disorders may be fundamentally different from those of individuals with intact linguistic functions, there are conflicting reports regarding the specific locus of anatomical anomaly (Foundas, 2001a). Although no studies have yet found a common focal neural abnormality that can account for developmental language disorders, various **structural neuroimaging** studies have pointed to various anatomical and morphological anomalies in the brains of SLI children. Several of these studies are summarized in an article by Lane, Foundas, and Leonard (2001) in the May, 2001, issue of the journal *Topics in Language Disorders* that is entirely devoted to *The Neural Basis of Language: Current Neuroimaging Perspectives*. Some of the studies discussed in the Lane et al. article (e.g., Gauger, Lombardino, & Leonard, 1997; Plante, 1991; Plante, Swisher, Vance, & Rapcsak, 1991; Preis, Jancke, Schittler, Huang, & Steinmetz, 1998) have indicated **atypical asymmetry patterns** in individuals with SLI—in other words, a tendency for certain structures to be larger in the right hemisphere than in the left hemisphere. This is particularly true of structures in an area of the **dominant hemisphere** known as the **perisylvian area** (i.e., around the sylvian fissure), a region known to be involved in language.

To understand what these findings of atypical asymmetry might mean, a brief review of the anatomy and physiology of the region of interest is in order. The major neurological components of language are located in the perisylvian area in the dominant hemisphere. It is important to note that by *dominant hemisphere* for language, we are generally referring to the *left* hemisphere. Ninety percent of the population is right-handed, and of those, 95% are left-dominant for language (Annett, 1985; Gauger et al., 1997). Even in the 10% of the population who are left-handed, estimates indicate that two thirds are still **left-hemisphere dominant** for language. The remaining 7% to 8% of left- and right-handers who are not left-hemisphere dominant for language are either right dominant for language *or* exhibit mixed dominance—that is, language functions represented bilaterally (Gauger et al., 1997; Geschwind & Galaburda, 1985). The point is that the vast majority of the population is left-hemisphere dominant for language functions.

Within the perisylvian area, there are several areas of interest with which most SLPs are quite familiar. **Broca's area** is in the frontal lobe and is responsible for many aspects of expressive language (e.g., motor movements, grammaticality). Heschl's gyrus, which constitutes the primary auditory cortex, is located on the superior surface of the sylvian fissure and is responsible for the conscious perception of auditory stimuli. Posterior to Heschl's gyrus on the lower, or horizontal, bank of the sylvian fissure is the **planum temporale** (PT). The PT and the lateral and inferior parts of the superior temporal gyrus form the core of **Wernicke's area**, which is responsible for comprehension of spoken and written language (Gauger et al., 1997; Luria, 1966). Numerous imaging studies have shown the PT to be typically larger in the left hemisphere. In

1968 Geschwind and Levitsky were some of the first researchers to suggest that the predominant leftward asymmetry of the PT is consistent with "known functional asymmetries" and therefore, may "represent the neuroanatomical substrate for language" (Foundas, 2001b). Interestingly, Foundas (2001b) notes that asymmetry of speech-language–related cortex has been found to be present in the fetus, suggesting that the human brain may have a "biologically determined, preprogrammed anatomical substrate for asymmetric representation of speech-language functions."

In summary, given current evidence, it would appear that interhemispherical asymmetry (i.e., larger size of the PT) is most likely associated with **language dominance** in that hemisphere (Gauger et al., 1997). Put another way, for the majority of individuals who are right-handed (and thus left-hemisphere dominant for language), you would expect asymmetry in the form of a larger PT in the left hemisphere. Lack of this asymmetry (i.e., PT *not* larger in the left hemisphere) would be considered anomalous, perhaps indicating atypical right dominance or lack of dominance for language (Galaburda, Sherman, Rosen, Aboitz, & Geschwind, 1985; Gauger et al., 1997).

The implications of this lack of asymmetry in individuals with SLI are vastly intriguing. It is unknown whether the asymmetry reported in some of the studies previously cited was the result of a reduction in the size of left hemispherical structures or an increase in the size of right hemispherical structures (Lane et al., 2001). Gauger et al. (1997) in their study of 11 children with SLI (using volumetric high-resolution MRI) discovered a difference in interhemispherical asymmetry for the total PT for these children (greater rightward asymmetry). In addition, the right hemisphere was significantly wider in these children compared with the control subjects, and the left pars triangularis was significantly smaller. Gauger et al. reported that abnormal asymmetry in their subjects was not due to increased growth on the right, but *decreased growth in both the right and the left hemispheres.* The authors speculated that atypical symmetry in these children might be due to *failure to establish appropriate neural networks for language functions.* Failure to establish appropriate neural networks might reflect disruptions in cell migration and axonal pathfinding resulting from either genetic or environmental causes (Gauger et al.,

1997; Leonard et al., 1993). Fibers that fail to make connections during the critical period eventually die and are pruned, leaving language structures that are smaller (Gauger et al., 1997).

Again, what might atypical asymmetry (as reported in these studies) mean for the SLI individual? Could this be the mysterious "neurological substrate" we have long been seeking as the underlying cause of language disorders? Unfortunately, the answer is still not that clear-cut or simple. But the new research does begin to shine a light onto anatomical differences in the brains of these individuals and point us in exciting new directions. Findings of atypical asymmetries due to structures being larger in one hemisphere than the other might suggest a different alteration in the course of development (Galaburda et al., 1985; Lane et al., 2001; Plante et al., 1991). Like Gauger et al. (1997) and Leonard et al. (1993), Lane et al. (2001) suggest that larger-than-normal structures resulting in atypical hemispherical asymmetry may be related to interruptions in the normal pruning process of neurons that occurs during early cortical development (i.e., corticogenesis). In addition, "dysplasias (i.e., abnormal growth/development of neuronal cells) have been associated with migration errors, while smaller than normal structures may suggest an interruption in proliferation or an extended period of pruning" (Lane et al., 2001). So it would appear that we really must begin to focus on the potential causes of such disruptions in the normal cell migration and the normal pruning process of neurons during fetal development and/or early childhood.

Some researchers have already begun to speculate on the source of these disruptions. In a study conducted by Preis et al. (1998), the investigators examined 21 children with SLI, along with 21 control subjects matched for age, handedness, and gender. Reduced asymmetries were discovered in the 21 SLI children and were associated with an increase in the size of the right PT and a decrease in the size of the left PT. There were also differences in forebrain volume and the size of the PT, with the greater volume or size on the side of the control group. Preis et al. also noted that there were significant differences in socioeconomic status between their two groups, which led them to speculate that socioeconomic status may have had some negative impact on prenatal development and resulting brain size for the SLI children (these interpretations of the findings are purely speculative).

It is important to note that issues having to do with group comparisons, research design differences, and difficulties surrounding identification of the regions of interest to be scanned using the neuroimaging technology in the studies previously mentioned make it difficult to compare and interpret the data within and across studies. I have not attempted to detail these many methodological issues here (for further information on these issues, the reader is directed to the Lane et al. [2001] article and the original research articles cited earlier). Still, it is tempting to speculate about the potential biological, genetic, and environmental factors that might cause these neuroanatomical differences in SLI individuals in the first place. What could cause failures in cell migration, neuronal pathfinding, and making connections between neurons during fetal and early childhood development? And more importantly, for our purposes as clinicians, *what can we do about it from a remedial or intervention perspective?* This latter question will occupy a good portion of the remainder of this book.

Structural Versus Functional Neuroimaging

Up to this point, I have reported and summarized data from structural neuroimaging studies of the brain. Lest I mislead the reader into thinking that the state of the art has truly achieved greatness in understanding what is going on in the brains of SLI children, it is important to note that, as reported in the May 2001 issue of *Topic in Language Disorders* previously mentioned, there are currently *"no functional imaging studies of children with developmental language disorders at the present time."* There is a great deal of difference between *structural* brain imaging (i.e., instrumentation that examines the anatomy or morphology of the brain at rest), and *functional* brain imaging (i.e., instrumentation that examines metabolic activity or regional cerebral blood flow while the brain is actively engaged in some cognitive or linguistic task). Neuroradiological and brain-imaging techniques may be organized in the following manner, according to what they measure:

Brain structure/morphology
  Computerized axial tomography (CT or CAT scan)
  MRI

Electrical activity
    Electroencephalography (EEG)
    Evoked potentials (EPs) or event-related
       potentials (ERPs)
Regional cerebral blood flow (rCBF) or metabolic
    activity or physiological-activation states
    PET
    Single photon emission computerized
       tomography (SPECT)
    fMRI

The lack of functional neuroimaging studies in children has to do mainly with the invasiveness of some of the procedures that measure regional cerebral activity, such as SPECT and PET, which involve the injection of radioactive tracers that have not been approved for experimental use in children. Although fMRI does *not* require the use of radioactive tracers, the procedure is quite loud, and the noise interferes with cognitive and linguistic tasks requiring auditory processing (Kroll and DeNil, 1998). The procedure is also sensitive to movement artifacts, and this restricts the use of the procedure to tasks that do not involve speech output (Foundas, 2001a). It is hoped that future advances in functional neuroimaging technology will allow researchers to overcome some of the aforementioned obstacles, thus allowing us a window into the complexities of the SLI-LLD child's active cognitive and neurolinguistic processing. In the meantime, SLPs should continue to read and learn everything they can about the neural bases of developmental language disorders in children, because an understanding of the neural bases of these disorders will surely help to guide and shape teaching and intervention methodology. The preliminary findings from structural imaging studies have shown great promise, and there is renewed interest in finding out more about the neurobiological substrates for language disorders. We now realize that children with SLI-LLD do not have a unitary disorder but rather a **multivariate** one, most likely resulting from a combination of genetic, biological, environmental, social, gender-based, and a host of other interrelated variables. It is unlikely that any one of these factors alone is sufficient to cause a language-learning disorder. Perhaps a genetic or neurobiological factor (such as atypical asymmetry of a language-related structure) in combination with some environmental factor (such as low socioeconomic status) might be sufficient to trigger a language-learning disorder in a given at-risk child. Future studies will need to explore how these variables affect the brains of these children during fetal development and during the critical period of language acquisition (i.e., ages birth to 5 years or birth to 12 years in particular).

Summary

In this chapter we have looked at the relationship between memory, inferences, and the comprehension and production of narrative discourse. We have seen that narratives (essentially stories) are a linguistic universal, are present from ages 2 years through adulthood, possess a predictable structure, progress in a predictable developmental sequence, and provide a rich context for language analysis and remediation. We have also explored the process of inferencing, or going beyond what is literally spoken or written, and how inferential processing forms a critical part of one's ability to construct meaning. Children with language-learning disabilities appear to have difficulty with inferential processing and the narrative genre.

We have also examined exciting new developments in the field of neuroimaging. Results of structural neuroimaging are providing evidence of atypical asymmetry in the brains of children with SLI. It has been suggested that the source of this lack of asymmetry (i.e., failure to show larger-than-normal structures in the typically dominant left hemisphere) may be related to an interruption in proliferation or cell migration or an extended period of pruning during early cortical development. Therefore, our goal during language intervention may be to take advantage of whatever flexibility is present in the SLI child's neuronal system by building new connections between neurons during the remainder of the critical period of language acquisition. How to build new connections through a variety of holistic therapeutic paradigms constitutes the substance of this book.

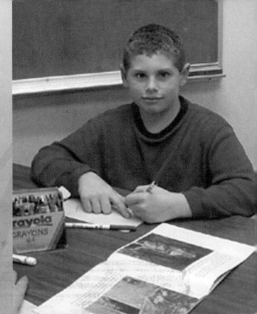

Chapter 2
Miscue Analysis as a Window into Language-Learning–Disabled Children's Processing During Oral Reading

Purposes

- Provide information on how reading miscues (i.e., errors evidenced during oral reading of narratives and other types of text) can provide a valuable window into the processing capabilities of language-learning–disabled readers.

- Provide forms for analyzing miscues by type, along with instructions for obtaining and analyzing oral-reading samples.

- Describe how miscue analysis can be used to formulate individual student profiles of reading and processing strengths and weaknesses.

- Discuss how this information may be used to plan language intervention strategies and to document the progress of treatment over time.

- Explore ideas for selecting and procuring appropriate children's literature.

- Explain how to obtain readability estimates for pieces of text.

Given the many potential causes of language-learning–disabled (LLD) students' or poor readers' narrative and inferential processing difficulties, it is imperative that teachers and clinicians identify the particular set of contributors for a given child and design instructional and remedial methods accordingly. The goal of any instructional or remedial method used with this population should be to teach balanced reading, or **strategic reading** (Trabasso, 1981). Strategic reading enables the reader to employ a wide variety of resources, strategies, and techniques to decode words and make sense of text and to generate inferences while reading. Discovering the source of inferential processing difficulties as well as the various strategies (or lack thereof) employed by a given reader is a complex task, however. Although we know that proficient readers employ a wide variety of strategies while engaged in constructive comprehension (Kletzien, 1991; Paris, Wasik, & Turner, 1991), poor readers may lack some or all of these strategies.

There is a tremendous amount of controversy in the educational literature about what constitutes a reading disability, the underlying cause or causes of reading disabilities, and preferred instructional methods for remediating reading disabilities. Some researchers are convinced that there is a great deal of **heterogeneity** in the reading-disabled population and that not all reading disabilities are alike

(Aaron, Joshi, & Williams, 1999). Aaron et al. (1999) point out that heterogeneity in the reading-disabled population is no trivial matter, because, "If all reading disabilities are not alike, depending on the nature of etiology, different remedial instructions may be warranted." The controversies surrounding the definition and etiology of reading disabilities may not be resolved anytime soon. Fortunately, in the meantime, a process known as *error analysis* (Kamil, 1984), or **miscue analysis** (Goodman, 1965, 1969, 1984; Goodman & Gollasch, 1980; Goodman & Goodman, 1977), can provide a window into the reading comprehension and decoding processes of good and poor readers and may be used successfully for diagnosis and intervention planning by those who have a more interactionist perspective on language-based reading disabilities (Lipson & Wixson, 1986). Specifically, teachers and researchers can hear the reader's departures from the written text (**miscues**) while the student is reading aloud and repeats, corrects, reprocesses, predicts, and monitors his or her own struggle to make meaning of the text.

In general, proficient readers are fairly successful at both **decoding** (i.e., getting the words right either covertly or overtly, by relating phonemes to graphemes [Aaron et al., 1999]) and at **comprehending** (i.e., understanding, constructing meaning, and making sense of what they read). The miscues that good readers do produce are fewer in number and generally do not grossly violate meaning. Poor readers, however, are often less successful at decoding and reconstructing the author's intended meaning. Subsequently, they produce more miscues overall, and the miscues they do produce often grossly violate the meaning of the text (Goodman & Goodman, 1977). In other words, their miscues are far from random, and much insight into the reader's process of making meaning may be gained when attempts are made to determine why the miscue occurred. Therefore, miscue analysis generally involves careful consideration of the type and general pattern of miscues exhibited by the reader. For instance, miscues may be broken down into two broad categories, such as **accuracy-related miscues** (ARMs) and **fluency-related miscues** (FRMs). ARMs include errors such as substitutions, additions, or omissions of words, phrases, or sentences and reversal of word order. An ARM may preserve meaning (for example, when the reader substitutes a synonym or semantically related term that still makes sense in the sentence) or may violate meaning (for example, when the substituted word is not a synonym or semantically related concept and does not make sense in the sentence). Although ARMs often signal that a reader is failing to decode and/or process the meaning of the text, FRMs may also reflect increased difficulty with decoding and processing. FRMs include too-long or inappropriate pauses; repetitions of words, phrases, or sentences; failure to pause appropriately for punctuation marks such as commas and periods; and inappropriate prosodic or intonational contours, including failure to elevate pitch and/or loudness for question marks and exclamation points, monotone or word-by-word reading, and an excessively fast or slow rate. FRMs may increase when the reader encounters a difficult patch of text, and although the reader may be successfully decoding the text and technically getting the words right, constructive comprehension (including drawing inferences and grasping subtleties of meaning) may not be taking place. For these reasons, detailed miscue analysis (augmented by question answering and other reporting techniques to assess comprehension) is an important first step when planning remediation.

The **miscue analysis system** shown in Figure 2-1 (DeKemel, 1998) is an adaptation and compilation of transcription and coding methodology recommended by Goodman and Goodman (1977) and others. It is designed to be used on oral-reading transcripts, in this case after children have read narrative-based or expository literature. The **miscue tally sheet** (Figure 2-2) is to be used to tally the various types of miscues and total number of miscues for each reading sample.

Subject Data: Oral-Reading Transcripts and Miscue Analysis

Before beginning a careful examination of sample miscue analysis data, I will provide some background information on the school-age students whose responses are used to illustrate various concepts in this chapter and throughout the remainder of the text. The majority of these data were collected as part of my doctoral dissertation, *Improving Oral Reading, Inferencing, and Narrative Abilities in School-Age Children* (DeKemel, 1998). The data were collected at two

MISCUE	SYMBOL	CODING PROCEDURE
ACCURACY-RELATED MISCUES		
Substitution	Dad / ~~father~~	Line drawn through miscued word; substituted word (including mispronunciation or partial or nonword substitution) written above misplaced word; phonetic transcription used when necessary to transcribe mispronunciations or partial or nonword substitutions
Addition/insertion	∧	Caret placed below line of text at point of miscue; added word(s) written above text
Omission	~~brown~~	Line drawn through omitted word(s)
Reversal	∽	Transposition marks placed around reversed words
FLUENCY RELATED MISCUES		
Repetition	R	*R* written over repeated word(s) (Note: Curved arrow used to indicate at what point subject reverted backward to repeat phrase; each repeated word in phrase counted as one repetition miscue) Ex: R̄ R R She's a very quiet baby.
Pause	℘	Elongated *P* to indicate inappropriate pause
Phrasing		Slash mark placed through missed punctuation
Intonation	↑↓	Inappropriate intonational rise or fall marked with arrows
Word-by-word reading	on time	Underlined word(s) read word by word
OTHER NOTATIONS (these deviations from the text will *not* be counted as errors)		
Dialectal variation	Ⓓ	Circled *D* placed above the miscue attributed to dialect
Self-correction	SC	*SC* written above and to right of another error notation, to indicate that reader self-corrected Ex: Dad/SC ~~Father~~

Figure 2-1 Miscue Analysis System.

elementary schools in Jefferson Parish Public Schools, a suburban school district that is part of the New Orleans greater metropolitan area.

The three subjects whose data appear in this text (Subjects 1, 2, and 3) were three members of a larger group of 12 subjects from the original study (six LLD subjects, six normal control subjects). Data from these three particular subjects were selected for illustration in this text in order to (1) highlight differences between LLD students (specifically, Subjects 2 and 3—two fifth-grade–age LLD students reading at approximately second- to third-grade level) and a normal language reading-age–matched peer (Subject 1, a regular-education, second-grade student); and (2) delineate qualitative differences in patterns and profiles of responses between the two LLD subjects.

Subject 1 was a regular-education second-grade student (white female, age 8 years, 5 months; socioeconomic status low- to middle-income). Testing revealed normal language abilities (total language score of 115 (mean = 100, standard deviation = ±15) on the *Clinical Evaluation of Language Fundamentals—3*). The girl was reading at grade level for her age (i.e., mid to late second-grade level) according to teacher estimates and according to the *Basic Reading Inventory*.

Subject 2 was a white female, age 11 years, 2 months, enrolled in a self-contained special-education class for learning-disabled students (socioeconomic status low- to middle-income). She also received speech-language therapy twice a week for a language disorder. Testing revealed severe language deficits (total language score of 54 on the *Clinical Evaluation*

MISCUE TALLY SHEET

Name: _____   Date: _____

Time Elapsed _____   Rate = _____ (words per minute)

ACCURACY-RELATED MISCUES (ARMs)   _____ TOTAL

_____ Substitutions   _____ Omissions
_____ Additions/insertions   _____ Reversals

FLUENCY-RELATED MISCUES (FRMs)   _____ TOTAL

_____ Repetitions   _____ Phrasing
_____ Intonation   _____ Pauses
_____ Word-by-word reading

OTHER NOTATIONS

_____ Dialectal variations   _____ Self-corrections

TOTAL NO. OF MISCUES IN PASSAGE (ARMs + FRMs) = _____

Ratio of number of miscues to number of words in passage (divide total miscues by total words in passage and multiply by 100 to obtain percentage) _____

$$\frac{\text{Number of ARMs}}{\text{Total number of miscues}} = \text{---} \times 100 = \text{---} \ \% \ \textbf{ARMs}$$

$$\frac{\text{Number of FRMs}}{\text{Total number of miscues}} = \text{---} \times 100 = \text{---} \ \% \ \textbf{FRMs}$$

Comments:
_____
_____
_____
_____

Figure 2-2 Miscue Tally Sheet.

---

of Language Fundamentals—3). Her instructional reading grade level was judged to be at the second- to early third-grade level, based on teacher estimates and results of the *Basic Reading Inventory*.

Subject 3 was an African American male, age 11 years, 8 months, enrolled in a self-contained special-education class for learning-disabled students (socio-economic status low- to middle-income). Subject 3 also received speech-language therapy twice a week for a language disorder. Testing revealed moderate language deficits (total language score of 75 on the *Clinical Evaluation of Language Fundamentals—3*). Subject 3's instructional reading grade level was judged to be at the early third-grade level, based on teacher estimates and the *Basic Reading Inventory*.

All three subjects received scores within normal limits on the *Test of Nonverbal Intelligence*. All three subjects passed a vision and hearing screening before participation in the study.

Directions given orally to the subjects in order to elicit the oral-reading samples were as follows:

I'd like you to read this story to me out loud. If you come to a word you don't know, try your best to figure it out, and then go on. When you are finished reading the story, I will ask you some questions to see how well you understood the story, and I will also ask you to tell it back to me in your own words, to see how much you remember. You may begin reading when ready.

No assistance was provided to the child while reading. If the child got stuck on a word and could not successfully decode, after a period of 5 seconds the examiner would say, "You may skip that word and go on." The readings were tape-recorded and videotaped for later transcription and miscue analysis.

The next section contains actual data from the three subjects in the form of oral-reading transcripts for the story *Jim's Trumpet* (Cowley, 1996) (with the students' actual oral-reading miscues recorded on the transcripts) and miscue tally sheets, followed by a section analyzing each student's error patterns and a discussion of how this information is relevant for intervention planning.

Reader Profiles Based on Oral-Reading Miscue Analysis

Subject 1: Normal Reader Profile

As can be seen from her oral-reading transcript (Figure 2-3) and miscue tally sheet (Figure 2-4), Subject 1 produced a fairly accurate reading of the passage; she evidenced a total of 22 miscues during

---

Story: *Jim's Trumpet*

Every night, Jim sat on the fire escape and played his trumpet for the little people in the building. He played eating music and laughing music. He played music for jumping and music for dancing. Then he played soft music for sleeping.

Jim was the <u>little</u> <u>people</u>'s friend, but there were two big people who didn't like the trumpet music. "Stop that noise!" they yelled.

"It isn't noise," said Jim. "It's music."

"It's noise!" yelled the big people. "Stop it at once!"

"I can't stop playing my trumpet," said Jim. "I'll just have to go and live with my sister."

So he went away to another part of town. That night, the building was quiet. No one could get to sleep. The two big people were awake all night.

In the morning the two big people went to see Jim at his sister's place. "We were wrong about your trumpet," they said. "You don't make noise. You make music, and we miss it. Please, come back!" So Jim came back.

When night came, there he was on the fire escape, playing music for eating and laughing and jumping and dancing. All the little people cheered and clapped . . . and so did the two big people.

Figure 2-3 Oral-Reading Transcript and Miscue Analysis: Subject 1. (Source: *Jim's Trumpet*, by J. Cowley, 1996, Bothell, WA: Wright Group.)

MISCUE TALLY SHEET

Time Elapsed: 2:25 (145 seconds)

$$\text{Rate} = \frac{\text{Number of words}}{\text{Time}} = \frac{206}{145} = 1.4206 \times 60 = 85.24 \text{ (words per minute)}$$

Note: To calculate reading rate or words per minute, count total time elapsed in *seconds* it took subject to read the passage (e.g., 2 minutes, 25 seconds, or 145 seconds); divide total number of words in passage (206) by time elapsed in seconds (145), which yields 1.4206; then multiply by 60 to obtain words per minute (85.24).

ACCURACY-RELATED MISCUES (ARMs)   ___7___ TOTAL

___5___ Substitutions   ___0___ Omissions

___2___ Additions/insertions   ___0___ Reversals

FLUENCY-RELATED MISCUES (FRMs)   ___15___ TOTAL

___11___ Repetitions   ___0___ Phrasing

___1___ Intonation   ___1___ Pauses

___2___ Word-by-word reading

OTHER NOTATIONS

___0___ Dialectal variations   ___4___ Self-corrections

TOTAL NUMBER OF MISCUES IN PASSAGE (ARMs + FRMs) = ___22___

Ratio of number of miscues to number of words in passage (divide total miscues by total words in passage and multiply by 100 to obtain percentage)   22:206

$$\frac{\text{Number of ARMs}}{\text{Total number of miscues}} = \frac{7}{22} \times 100 = \textbf{32\% ARMs}$$

$$\frac{\text{Number of FRMs}}{\text{Total number of miscues}} = \frac{15}{22} \times 100 = \textbf{68\% FRMs}$$

Comments:

_____

_____

_____

_____

Figure 2–4 Miscue Tally Sheet Subject 1.

her oral reading of the story (7 ARMs, 15 FRMs). The most common type of miscue was repetition (n = 11); these types of miscues are often used as a means of verifying or double-checking the meaning as the child reads along, and they do not tend to overly disturb the accuracy or integrity of the passage. Several of the miscues occurred on **contractions** (e.g., *It isn't*, and twice on the word *it's*). It would not be unusual for a second-grader to still have a little uncertainty about this morphographemic construction. In Chapter 3, Subject 1's oral-reading performance is compared with her comprehension of the passage, as measured by her ability to answer factual, interpretation, and inference questions about the story, and her ability to retell the narrative in correct detail. Overall, her oral-reading performance, as judged by this miscue analysis, seems well within normal limits for a child at her age and grade level.

Subject 2: Language-Learning–Disabled Reader Profile

As can by seen on her oral-reading transcript (Figure 2-5) and miscue tally sheet (Figure

2-6), Subject 2 had a total of 17 miscues in the passage (5 ARMs, 12 FRMS). On the surface, this does not seem like many miscues, and indeed, Subject 2 can be said to be a fairly fluent reader (i.e., relatively few miscues present; appropriate prosody during reading). It must be remembered, however, that Subject 2 is nearly 3 years older than Subject 1 and is reading approximately two to three grade levels below chronological age and grade-level expectancies. The fact that Subject 2 reads fairly fluently at her below-average instructional reading grade level could be viewed as a strength of sorts

---

Story: *Jim's Trumpet*

Every night, Jim sat on the fire escape and played his trumpet for the little people in the building. He played eating music and laughing music. He played music for jumping and music for dancing. Then he played soft music for sleeping.

Jim was the little people's friend, but there were two big people who didn't like the trumpet music. "Stop that noise!" they yelled.

"It isn't noise," said Jim. "It's music."

"It's noise!" yelled the big people. "Stop it at once!"

"I can't stop playing my trumpet," said Jim. "I'll just have to go and live with my sister." So he went away to another part of town. That night, the building was quiet. No one could get to sleep. The two big people were awake all night.

In the morning the two big people went to see Jim at his sister's place. "We were wrong about your trumpet," they said. "You don't make noise. You make music, and we miss it. Please, come back!" So Jim came back.

When night came, there he was on the fire escape, playing music for eating and laughing and jumping and dancing. All the little people cheered and clapped . . . and so did the two big people.

Figure 2-5 Oral-Reading Transcript and Miscue Analysis: Subject 2. (Source: *Jim's Trumpet*, by J. Cowley, 1996, Bothell, WA: Wright Group.)

MISCUE TALLY SHEET

Time Elapsed: 2:29 (149 seconds)

$$\text{Rate} = \frac{\text{Number of words}}{\text{Time}} = \frac{206}{149} = 1.3825 \times 60 = \mathbf{82.95} \text{ (words per minute)}$$

ACCURACY-RELATED MISCUES (ARMs)   _5_ TOTAL

_5_ Substitutions   _0_ Omissions
_0_ Additions/insertions   _0_ Reversals

FLUENCY-RELATED MISCUES (FRMs)   _12_ TOTAL

_0_ Repetitions   _0_ Phrasing
_0_ Intonation   _0_ Pauses
_12_ Word-by-word reading

OTHER NOTATIONS

_2_ Dialectal variations   _0_ Self-corrections

TOTAL NUMBER OF MISCUES IN PASSAGE (ARMs + FRMs) =/   _17_

Ratio of number of miscues to number of words in passage (divide total miscues by total words in passage and multiply by 100 to obtain percentage)   _17:206_

$$\frac{\text{Number of ARMs}}{\text{Total number of miscues}} = \frac{5}{17} \times 100 = \mathbf{29\% \text{ ARMs}}$$

$$\frac{\text{Number of FRMs}}{\text{Total number of miscues}} = \frac{12}{17} \times 100 = \mathbf{71\% \text{ FRMs}}$$

Comments:
_____
_____
_____

Figure 2–6 Miscue Tally Sheet Subject 2.

(i.e., it indicates that she has attained some mastery over the **form** aspects of the language, such as written phonology, morphology, and syntax). It is later in the data analysis, when we examine Subject 2's question comprehension and narrative-retelling abilities, that we will see where her greatest deficits are apparent. In the meantime, however, more data can be gained by an individual analysis of Subject 2's oral-reading miscues.

It is extremely pertinent that all of Subject 2's ARMs are *substitution* errors (Box 2-1), none of which were ever *self-corrected*. Normally, substitution errors (particularly when the error is *not* semantically related to the target word) are particularly injurious to preserving the meaning of the intended text. However, three out of five of Subject 2's errors (miscues 1, 3, and 4) are semantically related to the target word (and even miscue 2 is a partial word attempt at the target word,

so it is phonologically related to the target and not just a wild guess or nonrelated miscue). The true cause of errors 1, 3, and 4 seems to be a matter of the reader's struggling with certain morphological aspects of the word. In item 1, the reader has omitted the bound morpheme (*ing*). In items 3 and 4, she has exhibited confusion about whether to add the bound morpheme (*y*) to create the adjective *noisy* or to just stick with the noun *noise*. These are not huge errors in the grand scheme of meaning, however, and the general meaning of the text is still preserved.

Interpreting what happened with miscue 5, however, is somewhat trickier. Perhaps the reader struggled with differentiating the graphophonemics between two similarly spelled words. Or perhaps Subject 2 read the sentence too quickly and simply substituted the first *qu* word that jumped into her head. Regardless, this error is *not* semantically related to the target word; it violates

Box 2-1 Subject 2's Substitution Miscues*

1. sleep/sleeping
2. noi/noise
3. noisy/noise
4. noisy/noise
5. quite/quiet

*Miscue/target word in text.

the meaning of the intended text, and the failure to self-correct is significant. The fact that Subject 2 read the sentence as "That night, the building was *quite*," instead of "That night, the building was *quiet*," and then did not catch the meaning-destroying miscue and made no attempt to self-correct, tells us that regardless of the original reason for the error, the student was not *reading for meaning* at the time the miscue occurred. When students are reading for meaning, they hear when a sentence they have read aloud does not make sense (i.e., when it contains an accuracy-related miscue such as the one described), and this often serves as the trigger for a repetition and/or self-correction. That is, the child often goes back and rereads the whole sentence or part of the sentence containing the miscue that didn't make sense and attempts to correct the miscue by replacing it with the correct word. Failure to engage in this kind of self-correcting behavior indicates that the child did not recognize that the miscue failed to preserve the overall meaning of the text in the first place. This failure to recognize meaning-destroying miscues when they occur, along with subsequent failure to self-correct, is a classic symptom exhibited by LLD children. It only happened once to Subject 2 in this particular oral-reading sample; it happens much more frequently with LLD children who are nonfluent readers who exhibit multiple non–self-corrected miscues and can be disastrous to their overall ability to construct and preserve the author's intended meaning from text.

To summarize, by looking at Subject 2's oral-reading sample and by analyzing her miscues, overall pattern analysis reveals her to be what may be termed a *type I reader: fluent reader with relatively poorer comprehension in comparison* (again, her difficulty answering comprehension questions and retelling the narrative are discussed in Chapter 3). She is quite different in her response patterns and strategy profile from our second LLD reader (Subject 3), whom I discuss next.

Subject 3: Language-Learning–Disabled Reader Profile

As can be seen by his oral-reading transcript (Figure 2-7) and miscue tally sheet (Figure 2-8), Subject 3 exhibited a total of 98 miscues (29 ARMs, 69 FRMs). Needless to say, this constituted an extremely nonfluent reading of the passage (i.e., numerous miscues, poor prosody). It is also interesting to note how much longer it took Subject 3 to read the passage (total time = 3 minutes, 21 seconds, yielding a reading rate of 61.5 words per minute). Subjects 1 and 2 (both characterized as fluent readers) read at much faster rates that were almost identical (Subject 1: total time elapsed = 2 minutes, 25 seconds—reading rate of 85 words per minute; and Subject 2: total time elapsed = 2 minutes, 29 seconds—reading rate of 83 words per minute). Subject 3's reading prosody was obviously adversely affected, as characterized by word-by-word reading that was prevalent throughout the oral-reading sample (for example, of the 69 FRMs, 33 were instances of word-by-word reading, or flat, monotone, staccato prosody). Much more information about Subject 3's overall strategies can also be gained by analyzing his individual miscues, particularly the substitutions (Table 2-1).

Analysis of the pattern of errors reveals that Subject 3 is struggling primarily with the *form* aspects of the language—that is, the written phonology (graphophonemics) and morphosyntax. The fact that he exhibits occasional self-corrections could be interpreted as a relative strength in the sense that he appears to be reading for meaning to some extent and seems to recognize (at times) that the miscue did not preserve the intended meaning of the text. Analysis of Subject 3's oral-reading comprehension (i.e., his response to factual, interpretation, and inference questions about the story as well as his narrative retelling) suggests that Subject 3 is what I will refer to as a *type II reader: a nonfluent reader with relatively intact comprehension in comparison* (again, the key word is *relative*, as his comprehension is certainly not within normal limits when compared with chronological age and grade-level expectancies). However, given how poor this child's reading sounds—that is, when the adult facilitator hears the multiple miscues, poor prosody, and obvious struggle this child goes through in an attempt to read the text—the fact that he is somehow able to access some of the deeper semantic and conceptual content of the story, despite his

Story: ~~Jim's Trumpet~~ *[James Tr—/SC]*

[James sit/SC] ... *[playin]* ... *[R]*
Every night, ~~Jim sat~~ on the fire escape and ~~played~~ his trumpet for the little people in the

[R R RR] ... *[he]* ... *[he long(laugh and laugh]*
building. He played eating music, ~~and~~ ~~laughing~~ music. He played music for jumping and

[R]
music for dancing. Then he played soft music for sleeping.

[Jame R a RR] ... *[R/SC]* ... *[friends]* ... *[how/SC]*
~~Jim~~ was ~~the~~ little people's ~~friend,~~ but there were two big people ~~who~~ didn't like the

trumpet music. "Stop that noise!" they yelled.

[R R no/noisy   Jame It]
"It isn't ~~noise,~~" said ~~Jim.~~ "~~It's~~ music."

[It]
"~~It's~~ noise!" yelled the big people. "Stop ~~it~~ at once!"

[R sc R]

[Tell/SC RR RR]
"I can't stop playing my trumpet," said Jim. "~~I'll~~ just have to go and live with my sister."

[he/SC]
So he went away to another part of town. That night, ~~the~~ building was quiet. No one

[R]
could get to sleep. The two big people were awake all night.

[R R]
[It was/SC]
In the morning the two big people went to see Jim, ~~at his~~ sister's place. "We were wrong

[didn't] ... *[R R]*
about your trumpet," they said. "You ~~don't~~ make noise. You make music, and we miss it.

Please, come back!" So Jim came back.

[ea—/SC]
When night came, there he was on the fire escape, playing music for ~~eating~~ and laughing

and jumping and dancing. All the little people cheered and clapped . . . and so did the

two big people.

Figure 2-7 Oral-Reading Transcript and Miscue Analysis: Subject 3. (Source: *Jim's Trumpet*, by J. Cowley, 1996, Bothell, WA: Wright Group.)

struggle with the **surface features** of the text, is something to be wondered at.

Analyzing the readings of students like Subjects 2 and 3 and comparing their response profiles with those of normal readers allows us to postulate the existence of certain subtypes of LLD/poor readers, based on characteristics such as number and type of miscues, presence or absence of certain reading attack strategies, and overall comprehension and narrative-retelling ability. (Box 2-2 lists possible sub-

---

MISCUE TALLY SHEET

Time Elapsed 3:21 (201 seconds)

$$\text{Rate} = \frac{\text{Number of words}}{\text{Time}} = \frac{206}{201} = 1.0248 \times 60 = 61.5 \text{ (words per minute)}$$

ACCURACY-RELATED MISCUES (ARMs)   __29__ TOTAL

__23__ Substitutions   __2__ Omissions
__4__ Additions/insertions   __0__ Reversals

FLUENCY-RELATED MISCUES (FRMs)   __69__ TOTAL

__28__ Repetitions   __2__ Phrasing
__0__ Intonation   __6__ Pauses
__33__ Word-by-word reading

OTHER NOTATIONS

__0__ Dialectal variations   __9__ Self-corrections

TOTAL NO. OF MISCUES IN PASSAGE (ARMs + FRMs) = __98__

Ratio of number of miscues to number of words in passage (divide total miscues by total words in passage and multiply by 100 to obtain percentage)   __98:206__

$$\frac{\text{Number of ARMs}}{\text{Total number of miscues}} = \frac{29}{98} \times 100 = \textbf{30\% ARMs}$$

$$\frac{\text{Number of FRMs}}{\text{Total number of miscues}} = \frac{69}{98} \times 100 = \textbf{70\% FRMs}$$

Comments:

_____
_____
_____
_____

Figure 2–8 Miscue Tally Sheet Subject 3.

types of LLD readers.) The profiles that emerge obviously do not hold true for every case, and individual children do not always fall neatly into categories (indeed, the heterogeneity of the LLD population could almost be said to be a characteristic of the disorder). Nevertheless, anecdotal data has for years suggested the possibility of various subtypes of LLD, and emerging research data (not only from this study but from others) suggest that it may be prudent to look for patterns in the behavior of SLI-LLD children (Bishop & Edmundson, 1987; Conti-Ramsden & Adams, 1995; Conti-Ramsden & Botting, 1999; Conti-Ramsden, Crutchley, & Botting, 1997). The identification of subtypes in turn may prove helpful in selecting a particular rationale for or approach to treatment, based on the cluster of symptoms or response profiles present.

Planning Intervention Based on Reader Profiles and Strategies

I advocate a literature-based intervention approach that is **holistic,** in which no part of language is neglected. Nonetheless, given the evidence just discussed, it should be apparent that each LLD child will have a pattern of strengths and weaknesses that must be taken into account when planning intervention. Indeed, it is the heterogeneity of children with LLD (an issue that we keep coming back to again and again) that makes this population such a challenge to

Table 2-1 Subject 3's Substitution Miscues

MISCUE/*TARGET*	DESCRIPTION
James/*Jim's*	Semantically related, graphophonemic error
tr/*trumpet*	Part-word attempt, graphophonemic error
James/*Jim*	Semantically related, graphophonemic error
sit/*sat* (SC)	Semantically related, morphosyntactic error, self-corrected
play/*played*	Semantically related, morphosyntactic error
long/*laugh* and laugh/*laughing*	Not semantically related, graphophonemic error, followed by semantically related, morphosyntactic error containing addition error *and*
Jame/*Jim*	Semantically related, graphophonemic error
friends/*friend*	Semantically related, morphosyntactic error
no/noisy/*noise*	Part word attempt, graphophonemic error, followed by semantically related error
Jame/*Jim*	Semantically related, graphophonemic error
it/*it's*	Morphosyntactic error
it/*it's*	Morphosyntactic error
tell/*I'll*	Not semantically related, graphophonemic error
he/*the* (SC)	Not semantically related, graphophonemic error, self-corrected
at/*it*	Not semantically related, graphophonemic error
his/*was*/SC	Not semantically related, graphophonemic error, self-corrected
didn't/*don't*	Morphosyntactic error
ea/*eating* (SC)	Part-word attempt, graphophonemic error, self-corrected

SC, Self-corrected.

work with. At a minimum, we can look for patterns or profiles of behavior like those outlined earlier, but we must always realize that even within a profile or pattern there will be a great deal of individual variability. Nevertheless, identification of a pattern or a profile does allow us to make some basic assumptions about where to get started in therapy, as long as we keep in mind that intervention and educational planning should *always* be fine-tuned as we get to know our students better over time.

So, let us assume for a moment that we have a type I reader like Subject 2 from our data sample. How might we initially plan intervention for such a child? As you may recall, this profile is defined as a "fluent reader with poorer comprehension in comparison." A child like Subject 2 has attained some mastery over the form, or surface, aspects of the print (i.e., the phonology, the morphosyntax, and conventions of print such as punctuation and capitalization) but is still failing to access the deep structure or content or semantic aspects of the text. It is also possible that a type I reader, despite the fact that he or she has mastered the surface aspects well enough to produce them fluently in the oral-reading modality, may be unable to **integrate** those form aspects with **content** or **meaning**. In other words, if the adult facilitator

asks, "What does an exclamation point mean?" or "Why do you think the author used an exclamation point at the end of that sentence?", a student such as Subject 2 may be incapable of providing a plausible response, since answering these types of questions requires *integrating form aspects with meaning.* The goals of intervention with a type I reader should therefore include the following:

- Helping the reader discover the deep or structural meaning or content aspects of the text (by liberal use of scaffolding strategies [see Chapter 4 for a definition of scaffolding] such as preparatory sets, constituent questions, summarizing, and paraphrasing [see Chapter 4 for a more in depth discussion])
- Focusing on **lexical acquisition** and discovering the meaning of new vocabulary or concepts embedded in the meaningful context of a story
- Helping the reader integrate form or surface structures with content or meaning aspects (specifically, helping the child explore *how* and *why* the author uses specific grammatical structures and surface features to create meaningful sentences, paragraphs, and wholes)

Box 2-2 Possible Subtypes of Language-Learning–Disabled or Poor Readers

Type I: Fluent Readers With Relatively Poor Comprehension in Comparison

- Adequate decoding or word recognition (fluent reader, few miscues, miscues may be self-corrected)
- Reading comprehension much poorer in comparison with decoding or word attack ability
- Difficulty with content or deep or meaning aspects of language (i.e., semantics, concept formation)
- Better at form or surface aspects of language (i.e., morphosyntax, phonology)
- Narratives, although longer, may be poor in organization and cohesion (may ramble, provide nonsalient details while omitting salient information—there is a lot there but little of it makes sense)
- Spoken discourse: may be more talkative in general
- Difficulty planning and structuring discourse; off-topic or tangentially related comments, word-finding difficulties and circumlocutions may be present

Type II: Nonfluent Readers With Relatively Fair Comprehension in Comparison

- Poor decoding or word recognition abilities (i.e., poor fluency when reading; multiple miscues, miscues may not be self-corrected)
- Reading comprehension somewhat better in comparison with decoding or word attack ability (although by no means normal in comparison with age or grade-level—matched peers).
- Difficulty with form or surface or structural aspects of language (i.e., phonology, morphosyntax)
- Better at content or deep or meaning aspects of language (i.e., semantics, conceptual information)
- Although shorter in length, their narratives may contain the *essential* information relayed in correct temporal order (bare-bones narrative, i.e., there is not much there, but what *is* there makes sense)
- Spoken discourse: May be less talkative; failure to initiate and maintain topics; short, unelaborated utterances

Type III: Mixed Readers

- Mixed characteristics of groups 1 and 2 (e.g., may have poor decoding and poor comprehension)
- Spoken discourse: may display characteristics of either type I or type II, or both (i.e., low receptive and expressive abilities; weak in form, content, and use aspects of language)
- Nonverbal IQ testing may reveal borderline results (i.e., low-average to just barely within normal limits range)

- Focusing consistently on *comprehension* of the author's intended meaning as the goal and purpose of reading (and not just on getting the words right)
- Focusing consistently on **cohesion, temporality,** and **causality** (e.g., explaining *why* and *how* actions and events occur in stories, explaining character motives, describing the salient details while omitting extraneous details and nonsalient information) during narrative comprehension and narrative-retelling tasks

Let us now suppose that we have a type II "nonfluent reader with intact comprehension in comparison," such as Subject 3 from the data previously described. How might initial intervention planning for this child differ from that for a type I reader?

First, it must be remembered that this child is still experiencing significant difficulty with the *surface features* or *form* aspects of the language (i.e., phonology, morphology, syntax) as well as conventions of print such as spelling, punctuation, and capitalization. Content and meaning aspects, although stronger in comparison with form aspects, may still not be age and grade-level appropriate and likewise may not be integrated with surface feature aspects of the language. In the narrative telling or retelling domain, this child has a tendency to fail to provide sufficient information, and when talking, may not elaborate on answers or thoughts. Goals for intervention with this child may therefore take the following form:

- A strong emphasis on helping the child master the form or surface aspects of the language (i.e., phonology, morphology, syntax) and the conventions of print such as punctuation, capitalization, indenting, and spacing. Although it is best to help the child see how these form aspects and conventions of print operate in **context** (i.e., during actual reading and discussion of authentic stories and expository texts), *supplementary instructional materials* may also prove beneficial in providing additional practice in the surface or form aspects of language as well as conventions of print. For instance, **phonemic awareness** exercises, dry-erase boards with colored markers or small chalkboards (for engaging in **invented spelling** and other exercises that involve manipulating words and letters, **syllabification, rhyming,** and other word and letter exercises); word games such as crossword puzzles, Jumble, and Scrabble; and a variety of educational software and CD-ROMS on the market that address the aforementioned skills are resources worth exploring.

- A focus on *integrating* form and surface aspects of language with content (i.e., emphasizing that good readers comprehend what they read, and that reading aloud smoothly, fluently, with a lively voice is often an indication that the reader is understanding what the author intended.

- A sufficient time spent helping the child understand the meaning of morphosyntactical structures and conventions of print, and discussing why and how the author chose those particular structures or conventions to create phrases, sentences, paragraphs, and meaningful wholes. (Hint: Keep some sort of grammar help book available so that you can easily look up formal grammar rules to explain things like, "What is a demonstrative pronoun and when or how do you use one in a sentence?" or, "What are contractions and how do we make them?" or, my personal favorite (this actually came up in one of my sessions with a group of fifth graders), "What is the difference between a colon and a semicolon?" (I knew the difference intuitively but could not explain the formal grammatical rule without a little assistance from my trusty grammar help book.) These sorts of "Everything You Wanted to Know About Grammar But Were Afraid to Ask" help books are readily available in the reference section of every major bookstore (look in the section where they keep the dictionaries and thesauri). It is beneficial for LLD students to see that even speech-language pathologists (SLPs) and teachers have to look up the rules of formal

grammar from time to time, and particularly useful for the students to learn how to locate and access such reference materials as well. *No therapy room or classroom is complete without a dictionary, thesaurus, globe, world map, atlas, and grammar help book*, and possibly some of the other reference books now on the market (for instance, I recently purchased a dictionary of idioms and metaphors to work on abstract language forms with some of my older school-aged and adult LLD clients). You may wish to purchase a children's dictionary and children's thesaurus for your younger students; I have them make the transition to the adult versions as soon as is feasible. Teaching our clients how to use a variety of reference materials (both hard copy and on-line sources) is an important part of language-literacy intervention.

- An emphasis on providing sufficient information to the listener or reader during narrative telling or retelling tasks (be sure to emphasize adherence to story schemata and story grammar structure).

- A focus on being more descriptive both in the narrative genre and during spoken discourse (spend time contrasting sparse, boring narratives or discourse with more descriptive, elaborated narratives or discourse and emphasize that the latter are more interesting to the listener or reader).

For type III students (who tend to have deficits in both form and content), all of the above goals may be applicable. These students tend to exhibit very individualized profiles, and the SLP or educator may decide to place more emphasis and instructional time on one or several components of language during a particular lesson, a given week, or a particular semester. Variables that affect intervention planning may include not only the child's profile of strengths and weaknesses but also the demands of the curriculum, the availability of materials and support staff, and the child's response to intervention and progress over time.

Measuring Progress Over Time

The miscue analysis procedures previously discussed may be used before treatment for diagnostic and baselining purposes, as well as during treatment to document and measure progress over time. The same directions are given to the student each time an oral-reading sample is obtained, and collection and analysis procedures are essentially the same as well (i.e., the oral-reading sample is recorded and the transcript is later analyzed for the number and type of reading miscues). With treatment, most LLD children show a general trend in the reduction of the total number of reading miscues over time. However, interesting patterns and trends may also be seen with respect to the type of oral-reading miscues evidenced by the child. In some cases, children who originally presented with more ARMs than FRMs show a temporary reversal of that trend (i.e., the number of ARMs goes down while the number of FRMs goes up, as the total number of miscues goes down overall). Eventually, there is often a balancing such that the two types of miscues are almost equal in number (number of ARMS = number of FRMS); yet again, the total number of miscues is much lower than it was before treatment began. The point is that there will be a change not only in *quantity* (total number of miscues) but also *quality* (ratio/type of miscues), and this must reflect some sort of change in processing strategies on the part of the child. The opposite pattern may also occur (i.e., a child who originally presented with more FRMs than ARMS shows an increase in ARMS and a decrease in FRMs with treatment, until at some point the two types of miscues become almost equal, while the total number of miscues continues to decrease overall). DeKemel (1998) speculated that children who show these types of qualitative changes (particularly a balancing pattern between the two types of miscues, ARMS and FRMs) with treatment may be evidencing a *balancing of processing strategies over time*—that is, a tendency to read for meaning and content while simultaneously showing an improvement in the ability to master surface and form aspects of print. This interpretation is purely speculative, however; additional research is needed to confirm that these patterns occur with any regularity in this population and to provide more information on what the data might mean (DeKemel, 1998).

Other signs of improvement to watch for in the oral-reading samples of students (besides the hoped-for reduction in the overall number of miscues) may include (1) substitution errors changing in quality from those that are not semantically related to the target word to semantically related substitutions, (2) an increase in the number of self-corrections (indicating that the student is becoming more aware that the miscues fail to preserve the intended meaning of the text), and (3) improvements in prosody, including less word-by-word reading and more lively inflection overall (particularly during reading of character dialogue).

As always, even during the course of day-to-day intervention, oral-reading miscues provide us with the best window into the processing strategies of our students. It is when we hear a miscue or series of miscues that we know we need to stop the reading and provide parsing and scaffolding to help the student process the language and intended meaning of the text.

Suggestions for Selecting Books

Some of the first questions SLPs or educators who are making the transition to literature-based intervention ask are, "How do I know which books to select?" and "How do I know what grade level a particular book is on and if it is appropriate for a particular child?" These are reasonable questions, and they deserve to be addressed.

First, how should one select books? There are numerous publishing companies that produce children's literature, and these and supplementary materials are available through educational catalogues. Not all the publishers produce materials that are well-suited for literature-based intervention, however. Without seeking to endorse particular companies or product lines, I do feel it is worth mentioning several companies that are extremely well-known in educational circles for producing books and materials that are in keeping with a whole-language philosophy and literature-based intervention principles. These books contain interesting plot lines, solid narrative structure, and wonderful illustrations! I also mention these books and materials simply because many SLPs who are new to literature-based intervention have no idea where or how to get started in procuring appropriate materials.

Wright Group/McGraw-Hill is particularly well known for their stages and grade-level series of children's books. These books, particularly the *Story Box* and *Sunshine* series, are appropriate for children in preschool through elementary school. Wright Group organizes their books into stages—for example, pre-emergent (preschool to kindergarten); early emergent (grades K-1); emergent (grades K-1); upper emergent (grades K-1, 1-2), emergent to early fluency (grades 1-2); early fluency to fluency (grades

2-3); and fluency (grades 4-5). SLPs or educators may order a hard copy of the Wright Group/McGraw Hill catalogue or browse their on-line catalogue at *http://www.wrightgroup.com/*.

Scholastic also publishes numerous children's trade books, nonfiction, and other educational and supplementary materials. Their products may be viewed on-line at *http://www.scholastic.com/sitemap.htm*.

SLPs and teachers or related personnel need not rely solely on graded book series for literature, however. Any book (fictional or expository), poem, magazine article, or other piece of text at the child's instructional reading grade level may serve its purpose in this type of intervention (indeed, a variety of literary genres is recommended), and it is relatively easy to determine the readability level of any piece of text. Help is as close as your computer keyboard. The SLP or educator might want to check out "Kathy Schrock's Guide for Educators," which provides access to Fry's Readability Graph at *http://school.discovery.com/schrockguide/fry/fry.html*.

Or, type in the key phrase *Fry Readability Graph* or *readability graphs* into your Internet search engine and you will get several hits related to readability graphs in general (the Fry Readability Graph is certainly not the only such instrument available, just one that is frequently used and familiar to many educators). The Fry Readability Graph works in the following manner (directions adapted from "Kathy Schrock's Guide for Educators—Fry's Readability Graph," originally adapted from Fry, E.: *Elementary Reading Instruction*, New York: McGraw-Hill, 1977, p. 217). First, the SLP selects three 100-word passages from the text (story, article, etc.). Second, the *number of syllables* and *number of sentences* for each of the three 100-word passages are tallied. Third, the numbers are averaged (i.e., the average number of syllables from the three 100-word passages is taken and plotted on the horizontal axis of the graph, and the average number of sentences from the three 100-word passages is taken and plotted on the vertical axis of the graph). The point on the graph where the two measurements meet represents the readability level of the passage (i.e., the approximate reading grade level of the passage).

It is easy to see the correlation on the graph between increasing complexity of the passage in terms of number of syllables and number of sentences and how this relates to the readability esti-

mate (and remember, the graph does yield only a readability estimate—ultimately, the only way to know if a passage is truly at a reader's instructional reading level is to have him or her read it). However, the graph has been shown to be fairly reliable at estimating the readability or grade level of texts, and it at least gives the adult facilitator a place to start in choosing texts that are generally appropriate for a given reader.

Yet another method exists for determining readability estimates. Most word-processing software can provide information on the readability level of a document or portion of a document that you can open with that software. In Microsoft Word, for example, after you have completed your document, (1) go to the Tools menu, (2) click <Options> and then click the <Spelling and Grammar> tab, (3) Select the <Check Grammar with Spelling> check box, (4) Select the <Show Readability Statistics> check box and then click <OK>; and (5) go back to Tools and click <Spelling and Grammar> (to do a spelling and grammar check). When Word finishes checking spelling and grammar, it will automatically display information about the reading level of the document. (Note: To locate more information about how to obtain readability scores on your MS Windows software, go to the Help window in the toolbar, click <Microsoft Word Help>, and enter a query for *How to obtain readability scores*. MS Word indicates that the readability scores provided are based on the "average number of syllables per word and words per sentence." On MS Word 97, both the Flesch Reading Ease Score (which rates text on a 100-point scale; the higher the score, the easier it is to understand the document or documents, with scores of approximately 60 to 70 considered to be fairly easy to understand) and the Flesch-Kincaid Grade Level Score (which rates text on a U.S. grade-school level) are provided.

The real benefit of access to instruments such as the Fry Readability Graph is that it makes it possible for SLPs and educators to avail themselves of the plethora of children's books that are rich in narrative structure and beautiful illustrations and to use those books for diagnostic and instructional purposes. Again, we need not rely solely on basal readers or even on graded series of trade books from publishing companies. This is of tremendous help to SLPs and educators who are subsisting on a tight budget. I haunt the bargain section of many popular bookstores in my metropolitan area (e.g., Barnes & Noble,

Borders, Books-A-Million, Half Price Books) and have built quite an impressive personal library of children's literature over the years with relatively small financial expenditure. I also make frequent use of the public library in my neighborhood and the university library (which is surprisingly well stocked with children's literature because of procurements by the education and special-education departments). And garage sales and thrift stores are also great places to find used children's books at bargain prices.

Clinicians have also asked, "Will I have to use the Fry Readability Graph or other readability instrument every time I choose a piece of literature?" The answer to this is, "It depends." If I am using a storybook for research, diagnostic, or baselining purposes (and accordingly I need to be relatively sure of the readability level of the piece of text), I always do a formal readability estimate. But I also find that after using the Fry Readability Graph for a while, the SLP or educator begins to get a sense of the readability level of books and pieces of texts just by looking at them. Therefore, in the course of day-to-day therapy and during general instructional activities, some of us have been known to simply guesstimate the readability level of a text when pressed for time. Guesstimating also makes it relatively easy when shopping to select quality books for particular ages or grade levels just by examining the pictorial content, as well as the amount and complexity of written text at the bottom of the pages.

In summary, even if you or your school district is not in the position to purchase a large number of graded series books, that should not be a deterrent to starting literature-based intervention. That said, however, it is my strong suggestion that SLPs and educators urge their school districts to begin spending some of their budget allocation on purchasing graded series literature from companies like Wright Group and Scholastic (including the oversized "big books" for the low-level readers or preschoolers in particular). The quality of these materials and their ease of use (i.e., the fact that the SLP or educator can be assured of the readability level when selecting books for a particular child or classroom) make these

materials a valuable instructional resource. Many school districts have an inadequate supply of language-literacy materials in general, particularly the speech-language-hearing departments (this is only a personal observation, but having worked in several school districts and in multiple schools, I have found that there is generally an abundance of articulation therapy types of materials in comparison with language-related materials). Rather than spending more money on cookbook-type therapy manuals, skill-and-drill picture cards, and the like, school districts should purchase quality children's books and supplemental literacy-based materials that can be shared by the SLPs throughout the district; this is an investment long overdue and well worth making.

Another helpful suggestion (if you don't have books and can't procure any in the short term) is not to forget to access your school library and the Title I, Reading Recovery, resource classroom, special-education, and other related service personnel in your school and district. I was once assigned to a school where the Title I person had an abundance of Wright Group and Scholastic Books at her disposal (big books in particular), and she was happy to loan them to me when she wasn't using them. I likewise loaned her certain of my personal therapy materials—it was a very good bartering system that worked to our mutual advantage and that of our students.

Summary

In this chapter we have explored methods for analyzing the oral-reading miscues of LLD children. These miscues serve as a window into the cognitive and linguistic processing of these children as they attempt to construct meaning from texts. The adult facilitator can use this information to discern patterns of processing difficulty in these children in order to plan appropriate intervention and later to construct various scaffolding techniques on-line (i.e., during actual oral reading activities) while the child and adult facilitator engage in reading and discussion of various literature and literature-related activities.

Chapter 3
Question Comprehension and Narrative Analysis

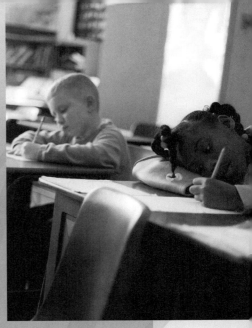

Purposes

- Discuss how to elicit and analyze children's oral-reading narratives for content, cohesion, causality, temporality, and adherence to story grammar constituents.

- Explore how to assess children's comprehension of narratives through analysis of their responses to a series of factual, interpretation, and inference questions about the story.

- Discuss how to use these baseline data for intervention planning and to document progress in therapy.

Sample Text

As in Chapter 2, the text of the story *Jim's Trumpet* (Box 3-1) is used as the sample text for the many forms and protocols discussed throughout the remainder of the chapter.

Baselining During Literature-Based Intervention

To obtain baseline levels of performance with the language-learning–disabled (LLD) child before therapy, the speech-language pathologist (SLP) should do the following:

1. Have the LLD child read a story at the child's instructional level *without* scaffolding and record and analyze oral-reading miscues (using procedures outlined in Chapter 2).

2. Ask the child a series of *factual, interpretation,* and *inference questions* about the story to assess comprehension (again, no assistance is provided during questioning). The SLP has to generate questions for the story and a list of acceptable responses ahead of time (Figure 3-1 shows sample questions for the story *Jim's Trumpet*).

3. Ask the child to retell the story (also without scaffolding) to obtain and analyze a **narrative retelling.**

   Directions to be given to the child during baselining are as follows:

   I want you to read this story out loud. If you get stuck on a word while you are reading the story, do your best to figure it out, and then go on. When you are finished, I am going to ask you some questions to see how well you understood the story, and I am going to ask you to tell the story back to me in your own words to see how much you remembered.

4. Tape-record and/or videotape the child's oral reading, verbal responses to the questions, and narrative retelling for later transcription and analysis.

5. Analyze oral-reading miscues using forms and protocols from Chapter 2.

Box 3-1 Text of *Jim's Trumpet*

Every night, Jim sat on the fire escape and played his trumpet for the little people in the building. He played eating music and laughing music. He played music for jumping and music for dancing. Then he played soft music for sleeping.

Jim was the little people's friend, but there were two big people who didn't like the trumpet music. "Stop that noise!" they yelled.

"It isn't noise," said Jim. "It's music."

"It's noise!" yelled the big people. "Stop it at once!"

"I can't stop playing my trumpet," said Jim. "I'll just have to go and live with my sister."

So he went away to another part of town. That night, the building was quiet. No one could get to sleep. The two big people were awake all night.

In the morning the two big people went to see Jim at his sister's place. "We were wrong about your trumpet," they said. "You don't make noise. You make music, and we miss it. Please, come back!" So Jim came back.

When night came, there he was on the fire escape, playing music for eating and laughing and jumping and dancing. All the little people cheered and clapped . . . and so did the two big people.

From Jim's Trumpet, *by J. Cowley, 1996, Bothell, WA: Wright Group.*

6. Analyze responses to questions and the child's narrative retelling according to the scoring system provided in this chapter (Figure 3-2). Sample factual, interpretation, and inference questions for the story *Jim's Trumpet*, along with sample data from Subjects 1, 2, and 3 (i.e., their scored question responses and scored narrative retellings) are also provided in this chapter to facilitate clinicians' training and practice.

Review of Subject Profiles

To review from Chapter 2, Subject 1 was a normal language, second-grade student enrolled in a public elementary school in a suburb near New Orleans, Louisiana. Subject 1 was selected as a reading-age match for the two LLD students (subjects 2 and 3). Subjects 2 and 3 were fifth-grade–aged students (reading at mid second to early third grade level) who were both enrolled in self-contained special education classes for learning disabilities. Subjects 2 and 3 were also receiving

speech-language therapy for language disorders. For a more detailed profile on all three subjects, see Chapter 2.

Analysis of Subjects' Responses to Questions

Subject 1

Analysis of Subject 1's responses (Figure 3-3) reveals adequate comprehension of the story. Subject 1 achieved a maximum 6 of 6 points on the factual questions and scored adequately (5 of 6 points) on the interpretation and inference questions as well, resulting in a total score of 16 of 18 possible points, or 89%. As indicated in the section on miscue analysis in Chapter 2, Subject 1 was a normal-language second-grade student (age 8 years, 5 months) reading at grade-level expectancies.

Subject 2

Subject 2 (Figure 3-4) did not score nearly as well on the comprehension questions, achieving a score of 5 of 6 on the factual questions, 3 of 6 on the interpretation questions, and 5 of 6 on the inference questions, yielding a total score of 13 of 18 points, or 72%. Although this is not an exceedingly low score, it is not what one would expect of a child this age (11 years, 2 months). As stated previously, this subject's instructional reading grade level was judged to be at approximately second- to early third-grade level (significantly below chronological age and grade-level expectancies). Although this subject's instructional reading grade level technically matched the instructional reading grade level of subject 1 (a normal-language second-grader), Subject 2 still performed more poorly on the comprehension questions than subject 1 did (a pattern that tends to be typical of language-disordered students; i.e., even if they are able to read a passage, comprehension tends to be poorer than for normal-language, reading-age–matched controls).

Subject 3

Subject 3 (Figure 3-5) achieved an overall score of 14 of 18, or 78% accuracy on the questions (slightly above the score achieved by the other LLD subject, Subject 2, but still markedly below the score achieved by the reading-age–matched normal-language peer, subject 1). Subject 3 scored 5 of 6 (83%) on the factual questions, 3 of 6 (50%) on the interpretation questions, and 6 of 6 (100%) on the inference questions. Subject 3's performance was very variable, and he seemed to process different

---

Student Name: _____   **Date:** _____

Story: _____

FACTUAL (score each 0, 1, 2)

_____1. Where did Jim like to sit at night and play his trumpet?
Acceptable Responses: on the fire escape; on the steps outside his building

_____2. What did the two big people tell Jim to stop doing?
Acceptable Responses: stop playing his music; stop playing his trumpet

_____3. Where did Jim's sister live?
Acceptable Responses: in another part of town; in a house in another part of town

INTERPRETATION (score each 0, 1, 2)

_____1. Why were the little people in Jim's building his friends?
Acceptable Responses: because they liked his music; because they liked the music he played for dancing, jumping, eating, etc.; his music was fun to listen to

_____2. Why did Jim decide he'd have to go and live with his sister?
Acceptable Responses: so he could keep playing his trumpet; because he wouldn't be able to play his music at his own building anymore

_____3. Why couldn't the big people and the little people in Jim's building get to sleep after Jim left?
Acceptable Responses: because they missed his music/trumpet playing; they were used to Jim's music at night and couldn't go to sleep without it.

INFERENCE (score each 0, 1, 2)

_____1. Why do you think Jim would rather move than stop playing his trumpet?
Acceptable Responses: because playing music is very important to him; he enjoys playing his trumpet more than anything; too much to give it up

_____2. Why do you suppose Jim's sister doesn't live in the building with Jim and the rest of his family?
Acceptable Responses: because she is grown up now and on her own; because she got married and moved away

_____3. What would you do if a neighbor was making too much noise in your neighborhood?
Acceptable Responses: ask them to stop making noise (like the big people in the story did); ask them to keep it down a little; ask them to play music only at certain times; call the police

---

Figure 3-1 Sample Comprehension Questions for *Jim's Trumpet.*

parts of the story with varied degrees of success. He seemed to have a good store of background or world knowledge to rely on, however, and this may have helped to elevate his score on this particular set of inference questions. His responses to some of the questions in the factual and interpretation sections revealed noticeable difficulty processing both literal and figurative aspects of the story.

QUESTION TYPE	SCORE	DESCRIPTION
Factual (F)	0	Inaccurate, incomplete
	1	Partially correct, incomplete, plausible but not probable
	2	Accurate, complete, most plausible
Interpretation (IP)	0	Inaccurate, incomplete
	1	Partially correct, incomplete, plausible but not probable
	2	Accurate, complete, most plausible
Inference (IF)	0	Inaccurate, incomplete
	1	Partially correct, incomplete, plausible but not probable
	2	Accurate, complete, most plausible

Factual question: Question for which the answer is explicitly stated or depicted in the text.

Interpretation question: Question for which the answer is implied or hinted at in the text but not explicitly stated or depicted.

Inference question: Question for which the answer may be neither implied nor hinted at in the text; reader must rely on background knowledge and reasoning skills to achieve the answer.

Figure 3-2 Question Response Scoring System.

Item Analysis

It is also useful to analyze the content of some of the LLD subjects' responses to the comprehension questions, for they are in some ways classic and typical of LLD children. Subject 2's response to factual question 3 ("Where did Jim's sister live?" Response: "In a house") is classically vague and nonspecific. Subject 2's response to interpretation question 1 ("Why were the little people in Jim's building his friends?" Response: "Because he made music instead of noise") is typical of a partially correct response that LLD children so often make. Subject 2 has understood the fact that the "little people liked Jim's music," but she has somehow erroneously coalesced this information with "the big people thought that the music was noise." This tendency to blur or coalesce bits of information that should otherwise remain separate in the reader's reconstructed version of the author's intended meaning is often apparent when these children answer comprehension questions about stories; this tendency appears to be yet another symptom of their overall comprehension difficulty (refer to Chapter 1 for a review of possible reasons for LLD children's difficulties with reconstructing meaning from text and their difficulties with blending and coalescing information).

Subject 3 gives his share of vague, nonspecific responses as well (e.g., factual question 3, "Where did Jim's sister live?" Response: "In a far town"). The substitution of "in a far town," for "in another part of town" (which comes directly from the textbase) is interesting and may reflect a word-finding error or other semantic difficulty. Subject 3 also gives several partially correct, or "almost, but not quite there," answers. For example, on interpretation question 2 ("Why did Jim decide he'd have to go and live with his sister?" Response: "Cause the two big people told him to get out.") Subject 3 gave an answer that was technically correct, but he failed to process the deeper levels of meaning that came from the **text-based clues**—that is, that Jim feels he must leave and go to his sister's house so that he can keep playing his trumpet, because his trumpet playing is so important to him. This deeper aspect of the meaning (which is clearly tied to character motive in the story) is lost on Subject 3, who at this point appears to be processing only the shallower aspects of meaning and coalescing them with his own background knowledge in order to make sense of that particular part of the story.

As with careful analysis of miscues, careful analysis of subjects' responses to factual, interpretation, and inference questions often provides a window into the clients' cognitive and linguistic processing, which in turn assists the SLP with the selection of appropriate scaffolding techniques and intervention planning. For example, if this had been a therapy session rather than baselining, the SLP could have

Text continued on p. 42.

Student Name: *Subject 1* _____   **Date:** _____

Story: *Jim's Trumpet*

FACTUAL (score each 0, 1, 2)

__2__ 1. Where did Jim like to sit at night and play his trumpet?
Acceptable Responses: on the fire escape; on the steps outside his building
On the fire escape. _____

__2__ 2. What did the two big people tell Jim to stop doing?
Acceptable Responses: stop playing his music; stop playing his trumpet
Playing the trumpet. _____

__2__ 3. Where did Jim's sister live?
Acceptable Responses: in another part of town; in a house in another part of town
In another part of town. _____

INTERPRETATION (score each 0, 1, 2)

__2__ 1. Why were the little people in Jim's building his friends?
Acceptable Responses: because they liked his music; because they liked the music he played for dancing, jumping, eating, etc.; his music was fun to listen to
Because they liked the music he played. _____

__1__ 2. Why did Jim decide he'd have to go and live with his sister?
Acceptable Responses: so he could keep playing his trumpet; because he wouldn't be able to play his music at his own building anymore
Because the two big people didn't like the trumpet. _____

__2__ 3. Why couldn't the big people and the little people in Jim's building get to sleep after Jim left?
Acceptable Responses: because they missed his music/trumpet playing; they were used to Jim's music at night and couldn't go to sleep without it.
Because they didn't have the trumpet to listen to. _____

INFERENCE (0, 1, 2)

__1__ 1. Why do you think Jim would rather move than stop playing his trumpet?
Acceptable Responses: because playing music is very important to him; he enjoys playing his trumpet more than anything; too much to give it up
Because he loved to play his trumpet. _____

__2__ 2. Why do you suppose Jim's sister doesn't live in the building with Jim and the rest of his family?
Acceptable Responses: because she is grown up now and on her own; because she got married and moved away
Because he's big enough to live on his own (Repeat/cue). Because she's bigger. _____

__2__ 3. What would you do if a neighbor was making too much noise in your neighborhood?
Acceptable Responses: ask them to stop making noise (like the big people in the story did); ask them to keep it down a little; ask them to play music only at certain times; call the police
I would tell them. Tell them it was too noisy. _____

Total = 16/18 = 89%

Figure 3-3 Sample Question and Responses: Subject 1.

Student Name: *Subject 2*   **Date:** _____

Story: *Jim's Trumpet*

FACTUAL (score each 0, 1, 2)

__2__ 1. Where did Jim like to sit at night and play his trumpet?
Acceptable Responses: on the fire escape; on the steps outside his building
At his house on the fire escape
_____

__2__ 2. What did the two big people tell Jim to stop doing?
Acceptable Responses: to stop playing his music; stop playing his trumpet
Make music/making noise
_____

__1__ 3. Where did Jim's sister live?
Acceptable Responses: in another part of town; in a house in another part of town
In a house
_____

INTERPRETATION (score each 0, 1, 2)

__1__ 1. Why were the little people in Jim's building his friends?
Acceptable Responses: because they liked his music; because they liked the music he played for dancing, jumping, eating, etc.; his music was fun to listen to
Because he made music instead of noise
_____

__2__ 2. Why did Jim decide he'd have to go and live with his sister?
Acceptable Responses: so he could keep playing his trumpet; because he wouldn't be able to play his music at his own building anymore
Because the um people said that you make too much noise so he thought, he couldn't quit playing so he had to go somewhere else
_____

__0__ 3. Why couldn't the big people and the little people in Jim's building get to sleep after Jim left?
Acceptable Responses: because they missed his music/trumpet playing; they were used to Jim's music at night and couldn't go to sleep without it.
Because he made so much noise
_____

INFERENCE (0, 1, 2)

__2__ 1. Why do you think Jim would rather move than stop playing his trumpet?
Acceptable Responses: because playing music is very important to him; he enjoys playing his trumpet more than anything; too much to give it up
Cause he thinks he needs to practice and make music and make people happy
_____

__1__ 2. Why do you suppose Jim's sister doesn't live in the building with Jim and the rest of his family?
Acceptable Responses: because she is grown up now and on her own; because she got married and moved away
Cause he made so much music (Repeat/Cue) because she's old to live by herself
_____

__2__ 3. What would you do if a neighbor was making too much noise in your neighborhood?
Acceptable Responses: ask them to stop making noise (like the big people in the story did); ask them to keep it down a little; ask them to play music only at certain times; call the police
Tell them um, "I like your music, I don't want to hurt your feelings but it's kind of making me confused and everything. It's good music and all but. . . ."
_____

Total = 13/18 = 72%

Figure 3-4 Sample Questions and Responses: Subject 2.

Student Name: *Subject 3*   **Date:** _____

Story: *Jim's Trumpet*

FACTUAL (score each 0, 1, 2)

  _2_   1. Where did Jim like to sit at night and play his trumpet?
Acceptable Responses: on the fire escape; on the steps outside his building
On the fire escape
_____

  _2_   2. What did the two big people tell Jim to stop doing?
Acceptable Responses: to stop playing his music; stop playing his trumpet
Stop playing his trumpet
_____

  _1_   3. Where did Jim's sister live?
Acceptable Responses: in another part of town; in a house in another part of town
In a far town
_____

INTERPRETATION (score each 0, 1, 2)

  _1_   1. Why were the little people in Jim's building his friends?
Acceptable Responses: because they liked his music; because they liked the music he played for dancing, jumping, eating, etc.; his music was fun to listen to
Because they cheered and clapped from when he played his music on the fire escape
_____

  _1_   2. Why did Jim decide he'd have to go and live with his sister?
Acceptable Responses: so he could keep playing his trumpet; because he wouldn't be able to play his music at his own building anymore
Cause the two big people told him to get out
_____

  _1_   3. Why couldn't the big people and the little people in Jim's building get to sleep after Jim left?
Acceptable Responses: because they missed his music/trumpet playing; they were used to Jim's music at night and couldn't go to sleep without it.
Because they liked all the music that he played.
_____

INFERENCE (0, 1, 2)

  _2_   1. Why do you think Jim would rather move than stop playing his trumpet?
Acceptable Responses: because playing music is very important to him; he enjoys playing his trumpet more than anything; too much to give it up
Cause he likes playing his trumpet
_____

  _2_   2. Why do you suppose Jim's sister doesn't live in the building with Jim and the rest of his family?
Acceptable Responses: because she is grown up now and on her own; because she got married and moved away
Um because she she was grown up
_____

  _2_   3. What would you do if a neighbor was making too much noise in your neighborhood?
Acceptable Responses: ask them to stop making noise (like the big people in the story did); ask them to keep it down a little; ask them to play music only at certain times; call the police
I'd tell them to stop doing it or I'd call the cops
_____

Total = 14/18 = 78%

Figure 3-5 Sample Questions and Responses: Subject 3.

followed Subject 3's response to the previous question with another question such as, "OK, it appears Jim has a choice. He can either stay at his building and *never* play his trumpet again, or he can leave all his friends and move to his sister's house, where he *can* play his trumpet. He chose to move away. Why do you think he made that choice?" Or alternatively, "Well, *why* do you think Jim would rather leave his building than stay and not play the trumpet anymore?" And finally, the clinician might query, "*Why* is playing the trumpet so important to Jim . . . so important that he'd rather *move away* than give it up?" These kinds of questions would stimulate further discussion and facilitate Subject 3's ability to process the deeper levels of meaning in the text.

General Suggestions for Generating Factual, Interpretation, and Inference Questions for Stories

The SLP will find that it is relatively easy to generate factual questions for stories, because these questions generally follow the pattern of *who, what, when, where, what kind, how many,* and *what color* types of questions. The clinician can simply scan the story carefully, examining the text and pictures ahead of time, keeping the aforementioned *wh* questions in mind in order to generate a list of factual questions for the particular story. Interpretation and inference questions are somewhat more difficult to generate, however, particularly when the SLP is first making the transition to literature-based intervention. It helps to think of these as *how, why, what if, hypothetical,* and *prediction* types of questions. Also, factual questions tend to follow the pattern of what the characters actually *did* in the story, whereas interpretation and inference questions tend to relate to underlying character motives, the more abstract moral of the story, and so forth. It is also wise to look for cohesive ties between sentences and paragraphs for potential interpretation- and inference-type questions (e.g., how one episode is related to another, cause-effect relationships). The boundary between what is an interpretation question (i.e., a question for which the answer is implied in the text) and what is an inference question (i.e., a question for which the answer is neither hinted at nor implied in the text) can be somewhat blurry at times; it is often advisable for beginning clinicians to create a

generic category called *interpretation/inference* to house any question that is clearly not a factual question, until more experience leads to a better understanding of the subtle difference between interpretation and inference questions. Note that this difference really has to do with the number of subtle clues found in the text (the answers to interpretation questions usually can be found as hints or implied clues in the textbase) and the degree of background information or prior knowledge the reader must generate to answer the question.

The SLP with access to a computer or word processor has the advantage of typing the questions and acceptable responses for individual stories and expository texts and gradually building a database that can be used repeatedly, modified, added to, and even shared with other SLPs. The building of such a database has proved to be a tremendous timesaver for me and over time has replaced many cookbook-type therapy materials, picture cards, and manuals.

Holistic Narrative Scoring Procedures

In the next section, narrative samples from Subjects 1, 2, and 3 are provided, along with a **holistic narrative rating form** and sample scored forms for the three subjects. The holistic narrative rating form provided (Figure 3-6) is an adaptation of several holistic narrative scoring techniques developed by Fox and Wright (1997) and Koskinen, Gambrell, and Kapinus (1993). The holistic narrative rating form is divided into two main sections: **obligatory features** and **optional features.** Obligatory features represent those features that must be present to form an acceptable narrative—that is, one that adheres to general story grammar and story schemata parameters. Subheadings under the obligatory features are (1) adherence to story structure, (2) major plot episodes, and (3) coherence. Optional features (e.g., formal beginnings and endings such as *once upon a time,* or *the end,* or evaluative statements such as "That gingerbread man should *never* have trusted that fox.") are characteristic of more advanced narratives, and thus additional points are awarded for the presence of these features.

The points from the obligatory and optional features sections are added to obtain a subtotal.

Subject: _____   **Date:** _____

Examiner: _____

OBLIGATORY FEATURES:

Score items 1-10 according to the following criteria:
0 = No evidence
1 = Meager to fair evidence
2 = Strong evidence

Adherence to Story Structure

1. Setting (indication of time/place, or implication of setting through other description)   _____
2. Identification of central characters   _____
3. Clear beginning   _____
4. Clear ending   _____

Major Plot Episodes

5. Statement of problem   _____
6. Statement of plans/attempts to solve problem   _____
7. Statement of consequences/resolution of problem   _____

Coherence

8. Correct sequence of events (temporality)   _____
9. Logical cause-effect relationships (causality)   _____
10. Correct use of relational and transitional terms, e.g., connectives (*and, then, so, if, because*);
deixis (*this, that, these, here, there, now*), anaphora (*he, she, they, him, her, their, etc.*)   _____

Subtotal _____

OPTIONAL FEATURES:

***Add** one (1) point to subtotal if present:*

Use of Stylistic Devices

11. Formal beginning (Ex: "Once upon a time"; "There once was...")   _____
12. Formal ending (Ex: "The end")   _____

Evaluative Statement

13. Metalinguistic statement concerning personal, world, or social significance of the story;
an abstract moral or lesson learned from the story   **Subtotal** _____

***Subtract** one (1) point from subtotal if present:*
14. Incorrect/erroneous information; addition of episodes or information not present in original story   _____

TOTAL _____

Modified from "The use of Retellings for Portfolio Assessment of Reading Comprehension," by P. S. Koskinen, L. B. Gambrell, & B. A. Kapinus, in J. F. Almasi (Ed.) *Literacy: Issues and Practices* (Vol. 10, pp. 41-77), 1993, Silver Spring, MD: State of Maryland International Reading Association Yearbook; and "Connecting School and Home Literacy Experiences Through Cross-Age Reading," by B. J. Fox & M. Wright, 1997, *The Reading Teacher 50* (5), 396-403.

Figure 3-6 Holistic Narrative Rating Form.

Finally, a point is subtracted from the subtotal if the narrative retelling contains incorrect, or erroneous, information (e.g., "Goldilocks stayed in the bears' house forever.") and/or the narrative contains the addition of episodes or information that was not present in the original story. The resulting *total score* constitutes the final score on the holistic narrative rating form. If an individual obtains the maximum number of points possible on the obligatory features section of the form, the total number of points possible is 20. If the individual also obtains credit for both items in the optional features section (and does not have one point taken off for the presence of incorrect information), then the maximum total number of points possible on the entire instrument is 22 points.

It is important to note that although this instrument has been used extensively by me, graduate clinicians in training, and practicing SLPs in Texas and Louisiana (who have been introduced to the instrument by means of presentations at various local, state, and national conferences), the information gathered to date using the instrument (other than the formal research project that constituted my doctoral dissertation) has been **anecdotal.** That is, SLPs have been collecting data with the instrument and reporting back to me in an informal way. Plans are currently in place to run a large-scale formal study with the instrument (in effect, to norm the instrument) with subjects of varied ages and grade levels from a large suburban school district in Texas. In the meantime, data from my doctoral dissertation and the growing amount of anecdotal data suggest the following:

1. Given the maximum score of 20 on the obligatory features section, a score in the 18 to 20 range is considered *high, normal,* or *good.*
2. Scores in the 15 to 17 range are labeled *low-average* or *borderline.*
3. Scores in the 12 to 14 range are considered *below average* (mildly to moderately low score).
4. Scores of 9 to 11 are *significantly below average.*
5. Scores of 8 and below are *severely below average.*

Analysis of Subjects' Narratives

Subject 1

Subject 1, the normal-language second-grader (who was reading-age–matched to the two LLD subjects), received a total of 19 points on the obligatory features portion of the holistic narrative rating form (almost a perfect score) (Figure 3-7). Subject 1's narrative retelling (Box 3-2) contained a clear beginning, middle, and end; identification of central characters; a setting statement; and a statement of the problem, plans, consequences, and resolution. Events were told in the correct temporal sequence, and cause-effect relationships (i.e., *why* things happened in the story) were explained logically. Only on item 10 in the *coherence* category did Subject 1 receive a score of 1 (for the presence of some revisions and false starts in the narrative).

(Although it is not specifically stated in the descriptive obligatory features of item 10 on the form, it became apparent during the course of rating children's narratives with the instrument that the presence of *revisions, false starts,* and *maze behaviors* [i.e., utterances that trail off and fail to end in the expression of a complete or logical thought; utterances that seem to hit a dead end, thus forcing the speaker to revert backward as in a maze to start over again before proceeding forward to express meaning] did in fact damage the smooth flow of the narratives [i.e., coherence]. Therefore a decision was made to reflect the negative effects of any revisions, false starts, and maze behaviors in items 8, 9, or 10 in the coherence category on the form. Future revisions of the holistic narrative rating form will most likely result in the addition of an item or clarification of an item or items in the coherence category [particularly as more formal data are collected on the quality of narratives produced by school-aged children at various ages or grade levels using the form]. In the meantime, SLPs are urged to use their clinical judgment and administer a score of 0 or 1 rather than 2 in items 8, 9 or 10 in the coherence category [whichever item or items seem most appropriate, given the particulars of the narrative utterance or utterances in question] when revisions, false starts, or maze behaviors disturb the overall smooth flow of the narrative.)

Subject 1 also earned some bonus points in the optional features section of the holistic narrative rating form; one point for including a formal beginning ("There was a boy") and a formal ending. No incorrect information or addition of episodes not present in the original story was noted (thus one point was not taken away from the subtotal), and thus subject 1 earned a total narrative score of 21. The maximum any narrative could earn on the instrument (total obligatory features plus optional features) is 22 points, so obviously subject 1 performed quite well overall.

To obtain a full profile of her abilities, one must go back and compare Subject 1's performance on the narrative retelling with her performance on the

Subject: *Subject 1* _____   **Date:** _____

Examiner: _____

OBLIGATORY FEATURES:

Score items 1-10 according to the following criteria:
0 = No evidence
1 = Meager to fair evidence
2 = Strong evidence

Adherence to Story Structure

1. Setting (indication of time/place, or implication of setting through other description)	2
2. Identification of central characters	2
3. Clear beginning	2
4. Clear ending	2

Major Plot Episodes

5. Statement of problem	2
6. Statement of plans/attempts to solve problem	2
7. Statement of consequences/resolution of problem	2

Coherence

8. Correct sequence of events (temporality)	2
9. Logical cause-effect relationships (causality)	2
10. Correct use of relational and transitional terms,	1

    e.g., connectives *(and, then, so, if, because)*; deixis *(this, that, these, here, there, now)*;
    anaphora *(he, she, they, him, her, their)*
    (Note revisions and use of false starts)

                                                 Subtotal   *19*

OPTIONAL FEATURES:

Add one (1) point to subtotal if present:
Use of Stylistic Devices

11. Formal beginning (Ex: *Once upon a time*; *There once was*)	+1
12. Formal ending (Ex: *the end*)	+1

Evaluative Statement

13. Metalinguistic statement concerning personal, world, or social significance of the story; an abstract moral or lesson learned from the story	0

                                               Subtotal   *21*

Subtract one (1) point from subtotal if present:

14. Incorrect/erroneous infomation; addition of episodes or infomation not present in original story	0

                                             TOTAL   *21*

Modified from "The use of Retellings for Portfolio Assessment of Reading Comprehension," by P. S. Koskinen, L. B. Gambrell, & B. A. Kapinus, in J. F. Almasi (Ed.) *Literacy: Issues and Practices* (Vol. 10, pp. 41-77), 1993, Silver Spring, MD: State of Maryland International Reading Association Yearbook; and "Connecting School and Home Literacy Experiences Through Cross-Age Reading," by B. J. Fox & M. Wright, 1997, *The Reading Teacher 50* (5), 396-403.

Figure 3-7 Scored Narrative: Subject 1.

Box 3-2 Sample Narrative: Subject 1

Story: *Jim's Trumpet*

There was a boy named Jim and he had a trumpet. And he used, and he sit, and he sat on the fire escape and played for the little people. He played for jumping, eating, laughing, and dancing. The two big people didn't like the music. So, they told him that it was too noisy. And so Jim, Jim, Jim said he was going to go live with his sister, and so he did. Then the next morning, they, well, they stayed up all night and then the next morning they came and, by his sister's house and they told him that that they missed they missed the music a lot. And then he came back and he played it for eating, and jumping, and dancing and sleeping. And everybody was happy and all the little children clapped and all the big children /k/, I mean all the, the two big people clapped. (Clinician O.K.) And everybody was happy. The end.

comprehension questions and oral-reading miscue analysis. As previously indicated, Subject 1 scored 89% on her responses to the factual, interpretation, and inference questions about the story (a *good* score) and evidenced a total of only 22 miscues in the whole reading passage (7 accuracy-related miscues, 15 fluency-related miscues; 4 miscues were self-corrected). Overall, Subject 1's profile is what you would expect for a typical, normal-language second-grader. She appears to be reading and comprehending at age- and grade-level expectancies, as evidenced by her ability to read a passage fairly fluently and her ability to recognize and self-correct some of her miscues when they do occur. And, perhaps most importantly, she appears to be *reading for meaning* and remembering a good deal of what she reads, as evidenced by her ability to answer questions about the story and her ability to retell the story in correct sequence and detail. No doubt these abilities will serve her well in the classroom, particularly when she is engaged in so many of the comprehension and production tasks related to the language arts curriculum.

Subject 2

Subject 2 (chronological age 11 years, 2 months), an LLD student enrolled in special education and receiving speech-language therapy for a language disorder, performed markedly more poorly on the narrative retelling task than Subject 1 (the reading-age–matched normal-language peer). Under the subcategory *adherence to story structure* in the obligatory features section of the holistic narrative scoring form (Figure 3-8), Subject 2 received scores of 1 on all four items (i.e., meager to fair evidence of the obligatory feature's being present in the narrative retelling [Box 3-3]). This means that although the information for the feature in question was not totally missing or absent from the narrative retelling, the information was by no means complete, detailed, or elaborated (which would be necessary to obtain a score of 2). For instance, Subject 2 failed to provide a well-developed beginning for her narrative, and her setting statement was incomplete as well. Although she did name the location of the setting (i.e., "the fire escape"), she failed to refer to the main character by his proper name, Jim. This is an important lapse, given that Jim's name is part of the title of the story and his name is used frequently and repeatedly throughout the text. Subject 2 *never* refers to Jim by name in her narrative retelling; she always refers to Jim using either the pronoun *he* or *the boy*. This use of a pronoun or definite noun without ever giving the proper noun **antecedent** is a problem in the area of linguistics, known as *indexing, referencing,* or **anaphora**. Subject 2 was also penalized for this difficulty with pronoun referencing under the coherence category later in the form.

Subject 2 also failed to provide a well-developed ending (her ending is rather brief and abrupt). She also failed to adequately identify all the central characters. In addition to not clearly identifying Jim, she did not delineate between the *little people* and the *big people* (she simply refers to *people*). She did mention "the um sister." A score of 1 (meager to fair evidence) for item 2 (identification of central characters) seemed to be an appropriate score, given these circumstances.

In the area of major plot episodes, Subject 2 performed much better, earning scores of 2 for items 5, 6, and 7. In the area of coherence, however, she again showed signs of struggle (particularly the aforementioned problem with anaphora). The presence of revisions, multiple interjections (*um*), and numerous grammatical errors or irregularities (e.g., "And so he came back from the sister, were happy") also tended to damage the overall smooth flow and cohesion of the narrative.

It is interesting to note some other peculiarities of word choice in Subject 2's narrative. For example: "and the people *close to him* said . . ." is a rather

Subject: *Subject 2*   **Date:** _____

Examiner: _____

OBLIGATORY FEATURES:

Score items 1-10 according to the following criteria:
0 = No evidence
1 = Meager to fair evidence
2 = Strong evidence

Adherence to Story Structure

1. Setting (indication of time/place, or implication of setting through other description)   *1*
   (Note: Subject named location, i.e. <u>fire escape</u> but omitted some of the setting/initiating statement such as how Jim played music for dancing, eating, etc.)
2. Identification of central characters   *1*
3. Clear beginning   *1*
   ("unelaborated" beginning)
4. Clear ending   *1*
   (brief, abrupt ending)

Major Plot Episodes

5. Statement of problem   *2*
6. Statement of plans/attempts to solve problem   *2*
7. Statement of consequences/resolution of problem   *2*

Coherence

8. Correct sequence of events (temporality)   *2*
9. Logical cause-effect relationships (causality)   *1*
10. Correct use of relational and transitional terms, e.g., connectives *(and, then, so, if, because)*; deixis *(this, that, these, here, there, now)*, anaphora *(he, she, they, him, her, their,* etc.)   *1*

                                                                                          Subtotal   *14*

OPTIONAL FEATURES:

Add one (1) point to subtotal if present:
Use of Stylistic Devices
11. Formal beginning (Ex: *Once upon a time; There once was*)   *0*
12. Formal ending (Ex: *The end*)   *0*

Evaluative Statement

13. Metalinguistic statement concerning personal, world, or social significance of the story; an abstract "moral" or "lesson learned" from the story   *0*

                                                                                          Subtotal   *14*

Subtract one (1) point from subtotal if present:
14. Incorrect/erroneous infomation; addition of episodes or infomation not present in original story *("sister and boy couldn't sleep")*   *-1*

                                                                                          TOTAL   *13*

Modified from "The use of Retellings for Portfolio Assessment of Reading Comprehension," by P. S. Koskinen, L. B. Gambrell, & B. A. Kapinus, in J. F. Almasi (Ed.), *Literacy: Issues and Practices* (Vol. 10, pp. 41-77), 1993, Silver Springs, MD: State of Maryland International Reading Association Yearbook; and "Connecting School and Home Literacy Experiences Through Cross-Age Reading," by B. J. Fox & M. Wright, 1997, *The Reading Teacher* 50(5), 396-403.

Figure 3-8 Scored Narrative: Subject 2.

Box 3-3 Sample Narrative: Subject 2

Story: *Jim's Trumpet*

Um, he um played his trumpet on the fire ecscape (dialect) and the people close to him said, "You're making too much noise." And then he s—he thought when he went inside, "I shouldn't quit playing I should, I think I should go to my my sister's house." So um, he went there, and then, cause the um sister and the um boy, couldn't, they couldn't sleep and so um the people that said you make too much noise came over. And then said, "Well, I'm sorry we thought um we were so wrong about it. Um (pause) you make good music so can you come back we miss it. And so he came back from the sister, were happy.

---

unusual way of describing the characters in question. It would have been much more appropriate (and typical) to say, "The other people in Jim's building said," or "Jim's neighbors said," or "The big people said" (using the terminology from the text). Referring to the *big people* as "the people close to him" may have reflected an instance of word-finding difficulty on the part of Subject 2 during the narrative-retelling task. (Word-finding difficulties were observed in other narratives produced by Subject 2 during my dissertation study and were also readily apparent in Subject 2's conversational speech and classroom discourse).

One strength of Subject 2's narrative retelling was the use of **character dialogue**, particularly inner dialogue that reflected the character's motives (e.g., "And then he-s-he thought when he went inside, 'I shouldn't quit playing I should, I think I should go to my my sister's house.' "). In future revisions of the holistic narrative rating form, an additional item (and additional bonus point) may be added under the optional features section for the presence of character dialogue in the narrative retelling, because this tends to be a sign of more advanced narrative development. In the meantime, the SLP should be aware that the presence of character dialogue in the narrative is a positive sign (indeed, it is something that the adult facilitator models, scaffolds, and works on during therapy sessions). The presence of character dialogue in the narrative retelling (particularly inner dialogue) may be considered as a sign of progress during treatment, particularly when it reflects the student's

emergent understanding of cause-effect relationships and character motives in the story. Likewise in the case of a student like Subject 2, the use of dialogue is a relative strength that can be used to bootstrap other weaker areas in her narrative.

In summary, Subject 2 obtained a subtotal of 14 out of 20 possible points on the obligatory features section of the narrative. No additional points were obtained for the use of stylistic devices or evaluative statements. However, Subject 2 did have 1 point *subtracted* for the production of erroneous information in her narrative retelling ("cause the um sister and the um boy couldn't sleep"). In the original story, it was the *big people* who couldn't sleep, because they missed Jim's trumpet playing. The subtraction of this point resulted in a total score of 13 points for the narrative retelling. As previously indicated, this score falls in the *below average* or mildly to moderately low range. By comparing Subject 2's performance on the narrative retelling-task with her performance on the oral reading and question comprehension task, one can ascertain that she fits the profile of a fluent reader with relatively poor comprehension in comparison. Although Subject 2 read the story *Jim's Trumpet* with a total of only 17 miscues (a ratio of 17 miscues to 206 words; 5 accuracy-related miscues and 12 fluency-related miscues), she scored only 72% accuracy on the factual, interpretation, and inference questions about the story (not a terribly low score, but not a very high one either, given the fluency and accuracy of the reading passage). Likewise, she received a total score of 13 on the holistic narrative-retelling scale (a *below-average* or mildly to moderately low score). Another way to put Subject 2's performance into perspective is to compare her performance with that of Subject 1, keeping in mind that although these two subjects are approximately matched for reading grade level, Subject 2 is *still* performing more poorly on question comprehension and narrative-retelling tasks than Subject 1 is (the normal-language, reading-age–matched peer).

Target of Intervention

The target of intervention for a Student like Subject 2 would be to help her delve more deeply into the meaning of the text. She has obviously mastered much of the surface aspects of the text (e.g., the graphophonemics, or sound-letter correspondences; the grammar structure of sentences; and word-formation rules). Subject 2 needs additional help with the following:

1. Understanding why *events* happen in the story as they do and how events or actions are connected causally and temporally (the use of a timeline as a graphic organizer supplemented with discussion of how one event triggers the next in the story is often helpful).

2. Understanding *why* characters act as they do in the story (e.g., character motives, plans, actions, and consequences). It helps considerably to perform activities such as connecting story characters and their dilemmas to real-life events or dilemmas and discussing possible outcomes and alternatives.

3. The deeper meaning of new vocabulary items encountered in the story (just because Subject 2 can read the words doesn't mean she understands them or how they are integrated into the story meaning as a whole).

4. Deriving whole-sentence, whole-paragraph, and whole-story meaning (i.e., the **gestalt,** or how the pieces, parts, and episodes fit together to form a meaningful whole.) This requires activities such as reviewing previously read pages more than once, summarizing, or paraphrasing.

5. Practice in retelling a narrative in both the spoken and the written mode (with focus on what listeners or readers *expect* when they ask you to retell a story and in what *form* they want the story told back to them.) Graphic organizers such as story maps and character maps are particularly useful in this domain (the use of graphic organizers is described in Chapter 4).

Subject 3

Subject 3 performed quite well overall on the narrative-retelling task (Figure 3-9 and Box 3-4). He adhered to the structure of the story, provided major plot episodes, and retold the story in correct temporal sequence. Scores of 1 were given for items 9 and 10, however, because of the presence of various factors, such as interjections, revisions, repetitions, and nonspecific referents, that disturbed the logical cause-effect relationships expressed and interfered with the overall smooth flow and coherence of the retelling. A subtotal of 18 of 20 (a *good* score) was obtained on the obligatory features section of the narrative. No additional points were obtained in the optional features section, and no points were taken

away for the presence of erroneous information or the addition of episodes not present in the original story. Therefore, the total score remained 18 points.

Overall, subject 3's narrative retelling sounded choppy because of the presence of the aforementioned interjections, revisions, repetitions, and so forth. Nevertheless, the essential information was present. When Subject 3's performance on the narrative-retelling task was compared with his performance on the oral-reading task and the question comprehension task, Subject 3 appeared to be a nonfluent reader with relatively intact comprehension in comparison. He scored 78% accuracy on the factual, interpretation, and inference questions (not a *high* score but not abysmally low either, given the struggles he exhibited with reading the passage), and his narrative retelling, although choppy and lacking in smoothness and coherence, did contain the essential information and macrostructure elements of the original story. Obviously despite his many struggles with the surface aspects of the written language of the text (i.e., the phonology, morphology, and syntax), Subject 3 still managed to extract and reconstruct a good deal of the author's intended meaning (although still not as much as a normal reader would, as evidenced by his struggle with some of the comprehension questions).

Target of Intervention
The goal of intervention with a student like Subject 3 would be to help him work on breaking the surface code (e.g., graphophonemics, morphosyntax) so that his effortful struggles to decode and get the words right would not hinder his efforts to reconstruct the meaning of the text. Again, helping the student balance strategies for meaning and form is the goal of intervention, and the result should be improvements in both fluency and comprehension. Much time and effort will need to be spent helping Subject 3 parse words, sentences, and paragraphs into their constituent elements, discuss formal grammar rules, and, most importantly, function at the critical intersection between form and meaning by asking and answering questions such as the following:

1. *Why* does the author construct the sentence in such a way, choosing these particular words in this particular order (and not some other order)? It is often helpful to change the order of the words around in the sentences from the text as an exercise, so that the student can see

Subject: *Subject 3* _____   **Date:** _____

Examiner: _____

OBLIGATORY FEATURES:

Score items 1-10 according to the following criteria:
0 = No evidence
1 = Meager to fair evidence
2 = Strong evidence

Adherence to Story Structure

1. Setting (indication of time/place, or implication of setting through other description)   *2*
2. Identification of central characters   *2*
3. Clear beginning   *2*
4. Clear ending   *2*

Major Plot Episodes

5. Statement of problem   *2*
6. Statement of plans/attempts to solve problem   *2*
7. Statement of consequences/resolution of problem   *2*

Coherence

8. Correct sequence of events (temporality)   *2*
9. Logical cause-effect relationships (causality)   *1*
10. Correct use of relational and transitional terms, e.g., connectives *(and, then, so, if, because)*;
    deixis *(this, that, these, here, there, now)*, anaphora *(he, she, they, him, her, their)*   *1*

                                                                    Subtotal   *18*

OPTIONAL FEATURES:

Add one (1) point to subtotal if present:
Use of Stylistic Devices
11. Formal beginning (Ex: *Once upon a time; There once was*)   *0*
12. Formal ending (Ex: *The end*)   *0*

Evaluative Statement

13. Metalinguistic statement concerning personal, world, or social significance of
    the story; an abstract "moral" or "lesson learned" from the story   *0*

                                                                    Subtotal   *18*

Subtract one (1) point from subtotal if present:

14. Incorrect/erroneous infomation; addition of episodes or infomation not present in original story   *0*

                                                                    TOTAL   *18*

Modified from "The use of Retellings for Portfolio Assessment of Reading Comprehension," by P. S. Koskinen, L. B. Gambrell, & B. A. Kapinus, in J. F. Almasi (Ed.) *Literacy: Issues and Practices* (Vol. 10, pp. 41-77), 1993, Silver Spring, MD: State of Maryland International Reading Association Yearbook; and "Connecting School and Home Literacy Experiences Through Cross-Age Reading," by B. J. Fox & M. Wright, 1997, *The Reading* Teacher 50(5), 396-403.

Figure 3-9 Scored Narrative: Subject 3.

and hear the resulting change in meaning that often occurs.

2. Why did the author choose a particular punctuation and style, and what happens to the meaning of the sentence or paragraph if you omit or change the punctuation and style? Again, showing how elements of form such as punctuation, handwriting, spacing, and indenting can affect the reader and alter meaning makes these small pieces and parts

Box 3-4 Sample Narrative: Subject 3

Story: *Jim's Trumpet*

Um, they had a, Jim was playing music for the little kids, in, in the building. He he was playing it on the fire escape. And one day, at night, the kids went to bed. And the two big people told the um, the ma—the—Jim that it was too noisy, go away and he went live with is sister. And that morning, no, and um when he went and lived with his sister the kids couldn't sleep and the um, bi-two big people was up all night. So that morning, the next morning, they went to um, Jim's sister's house. And um (Pause) asked Jim to come back and stuff. So he went back and um (Pause) play—he was playing music on the fire escape, and everybody and um, the little people cheered and clapped. The big people cheered and clapped.

suddenly much more relevant. Activities such as paragraph formulation, written narrative summarization, and the various planning, drafting, proofing, editing, and revising stages of the natural writing process are perfect for exploring how the elements of form and meaning work together; the student and clinician end up essentially deconstructing and reconstructing language, using the permanency of the written text as a facilitative context.

3. How do all of the elements—sounds or letters, words, and phrases—bind and blend together as a whole to create meaning?

Getting Started—Hanging in There!

SLPs who are beginning to make the transition to narrative and literature-based intervention often feel daunted and overwhelmed by a process and methods that just feel so different from the traditional skills-based approach to treatment that they were taught. This trepidation is normal. But do not get discouraged! SLPs and other educators and service providers should make the transition to the new methods at a rate that feels comfortable and appropriate. I have heard from many SLPs (after presenting this information to them at conferences and workshops) who have taken the time to contact me in subsequent days, weeks, or even years to update me on their progress as they make the transition

from skills-based to literature-based intervention formats. Many report that they got started by choosing just one or two of their language groups at the beginning or, alternately, by incorporating a portion of literature and thematic activities into part of each of their language sessions. Many others, after experimentation over time, have concluded what I have concluded as well: that literature-based intervention need not replace traditional skills-based approaches. Instead, in many cases, it can serve as a useful supplement or adjunct to more traditional skills-based approaches. In other situations, SLPs are finding that it is appropriate (given their particular circumstances and the needs of their students) to use literature-based intervention as their primary instructional and therapeutic format, with traditional skills-based activities serving as the supplemental format. Indeed, it is the flexibility of the intervention strategies associated with literature-based intervention (discussed in Chapter 4) and the flexibility of being able to segue from one therapeutic paradigm to another as we deem appropriate that has exemplified an area of tremendous progress in our profession during the 1990s (see Chapter 7 for more details). So much of the choice about intervention methods is now driven by (and should be driven by) the needs of individual clients. And the needs of individual clients are in turn based on our better understanding of variables such as cultural and linguistic differences, socioeconomic status, the individual pattern or profile of the language disorder present, classroom or curricular needs, parental or teacher involvement, and a host of other variables. Therefore, some of the goals for the SLP of the new millennium should be as follows:

1. Be brave, forward thinking, and flexible in trying alternative therapeutic paradigms.
2. Be open-minded about methods for measuring the progress of treatment and documenting the efficacy of treatment (the traditional plus-and-minus scoring of the past is not necessarily appropriate for the kinds of abilities I have been discussing in this chapter).
3. Take your time in making the transition to new paradigms (better to start small and focus on *quality* rather than *quantity* when trying out a new method or service delivery option during the initial stages). Success from small starts will breed confidence, and confidence will ensure continued growth.

Summary

In this chapter we have discussed how to obtain baseline data on students' oral narrative-retelling abilities, as well as how to assess their comprehension of stories by means of response to factual, interpretation, and inference questions about stories. These techniques (along with the forms and protocols provided) can be used not only to collect baseline data for students at the beginning of therapy but also to document progress in treatment over time. As students become more adept at processing both meaning and form aspects of language during treatment, scores on both the narrative retelling and the comprehension questions should improve. We have seen (through analysis of actual subject data) how performance on oral reading, narrative retelling, and question comprehension tends to provide a profile or pattern of linguistic processing for each individual student, and that this profile can then be used for intervention-planning purposes. In Chapter 4, I discuss actual intervention strategies for improving narrative and inferential processing abilities in LLD children, as well as techniques for addressing other form and content aspects of language.

Chapter 4
Designing Thematic Units and Measuring Treatment Outcomes

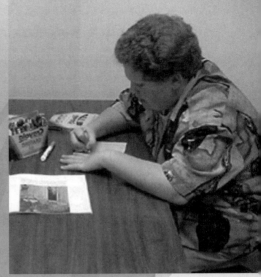

Purposes

- Review initial baselining procedures and link those with information on how to get started in therapy.
- Discuss how to design thematic units.
- Provide specific protocols, forms, and instructions to assist the speech-language pathologist in developing the thematic units, including lesson plans, skills and concepts to target sheets, story maps, and character maps.
- Provide sample excerpts from authentic literature texts to illustrate the building of thematic units and related concepts.
- Provide specific forms, protocols, and instructions for baselining and for measuring the progress of treatment over time.

Selecting Texts and Storybooks

The first challenge for the speech-language pathologist (SLP) when planning and implementing literature-based intervention is to choose books that are at the appropriate level of complexity for the language-learning–disabled (LLD) child. In selecting books, care should be taken to avoid books that are too difficult or too easy for the student. In general, the books chosen should be at the student's **instructional reading grade level** (i.e., books that the child can read without undue struggle or frustration, with adult assistance). Books that are at the child's **frustrational reading level** (i.e., books

that cause undue struggle or frustration, that result in multiple miscues, or that the child cannot read, even with adult assistance) or books that are at the child's **independent reading level** (i.e., books that the child can read easily, with few or no miscues) do not make the best choices for intervention.

There are many sources for appropriate literature for children, such as school libraries, local bookstores, classrooms, and the plethora of catalogues and publishing companies that produce graded series of children's fiction, trade books, and expository texts (see Chapter 2). It is possible to take any piece of literature and determine an approximation of its readability level by using a readability graph. Fry's Readability Graph, described in Chapter 2, is one such instrument that has been available for quite some time. In general, instruments such as Fry's Readability Graph require the user to count the number of words and number of syllables within a given number of sentences and to plot that information on a graph. The graph then provides a grade-level readability estimate (e.g., a passage of text may be determined to be at fourth-grade reading level).

Other readability graphs are available on the Internet and also on many word-processing packages such as Microsoft Word, as described in Chapter 2.

Box 4-1 shows the text of *Jim's Trumpet* (Cowley, 1996), which is suitable for a child reading at approximately second-grade level. *Jim's*

Box 4-1 Text of *Jim's Trumpet*

Every night, Jim sat on the fire escape and played his trumpet for the little people in the building.

He played eating music and laughing music. He played music for jumping and music for dancing. Then he played soft music for sleeping.

Jim was the little people's friend, but there were two big people who didn't like the trumpet music. "Stop that noise!" they yelled.

"It isn't noise," said Jim. "It's music."

"It's noise!" yelled the big people. "Stop it at once!"

"I can't stop playing my trumpet," said Jim. "I'll just have to go and live with my sister."

So he went away to another part of town. That night, the building was quiet. No one could get to sleep. The two big people were awake all night.

In the morning the two big people went to see Jim at his sister's place. "We were wrong about your trumpet," they said. "You don't make noise. You make music, and we miss it. Please, come back!" So Jim came back.

When night came, there he was on the fire escape, playing music for eating and laughing and jumping and dancing. All the little people cheered and clapped . . . and so did the two big people.

From Jim's Trumpet, *by J. Cowley, 1996, Bothell, WA: Wright Group.*

Trumpet is also an appropriate narrative for intervention purposes, given its adherence to story grammar structure, its lively and meaningful plot, and colorful and vivid illustrations. *Jim's Trumpet* is used as the sample text for the many forms and protocols discussed throughout the remainder of this chapter.

Baselining and Measuring Progress During Literature-Based Intervention

As discussed in previous chapters, to obtain baseline levels of performance with the LLD child before therapy, the SLP should engage in the following procedures:

1. Have the LLD child read a story at the child's instructional reading level *without* scaffolding or assistance, and record and analyze oral-reading miscues (as discussed in Chapter 2).

2. Ask the child a series of factual, interpretation, and inference questions about the story to assess comprehension (again, no assistance should be provided during questioning). The SLP must generate questions for the story and a list of acceptable responses ahead of time (see discussion in Chapter 3, which also contains sample questions and client responses for *Jim's Trumpet*).

3. Ask the child to retell the story (also without scaffolding) to obtain and analyze a narrative retelling.

Directions to give to the child before the oral reading and question and narrative elicitation are as follows:

> *I want you to read this story out loud. If you get stuck on a word while you are reading the story, do your best to figure it out, and then go on. When you are finished, I am going to ask you some questions to see how well you understood the story, and I am going to ask you to tell the story back to me in your own words to see how much you remembered.*

4. Tape-record and/or videotape the child's oral reading, response to the questions, and narrative retelling for later analysis.

5. Analyze oral-reading miscues using forms and procedures discussed in Chapter 2.

6. Score responses to comprehension questions and analyze the narrative retelling (further directions, sample narratives, and scoring protocols are described in Chapter 3).

7. Analyze and synthesize all baseline data, and form initial impressions of child's reading and language profile.

8. Begin therapy, using the same story as used during baseline, but this time, provide scaffolding as needed (these procedures are discussed later in this chapter).

In the pages to follow, various forms and protocols are presented for use in baselining and measuring treatment outcomes during literature-based intervention. These forms may be used at the beginning of therapy and intermittently throughout therapy to assess progress and to determine if changes in intervention are warranted.

After Baselining: Getting Ready for Intervention

Perhaps one of the greatest obstacles SLPs face in making the transition to literature-based intervention is that our traditional record-keeping procedures and paperwork (e.g., lesson plans, daily tally sheets, progress notes) do not fit with this innovative intervention format. Often this obstacle alone is enough to deter SLPs from attempting to make the switch to holistic, literature-based intervention formats. I have even encountered instances in which school administrators have set rules forbidding SLPs from using any sort of lesson plans or progress notes that do not follow the more traditional format (i.e., forms or record-keeping procedures that do not adhere to plus-or-minus or percentage-type scoring). Fortunately, the rules are changing, and most school districts are becoming more and more receptive to the idea of descriptive-type protocols such as those that are discussed in the next section.

Several years ago, I created a lesson plan format that, for lack of a better term, has come to be called the **skills and concepts to target** (SCT) **sheet**. The purpose of the SCT sheet was to impose some structure on what is often perceived to be a very loose and open-ended intervention format. This in turn would allow beginning graduate student clinicians to take a story or expository text and identify the various linguistic elements to be targeted during a literature-based therapy session with an LLD child. Many of these beginning graduate clinicians had had some exposure to traditional record-keeping formats in their undergraduate programs, and they were rather rigidly clinging to the notion that only behaviors that could be scored with pluses and minuses could and should be addressed in therapy. It was something of a revelation to these clinicians to discover that we target functional and appropriate language goals and objectives for LLD children (i.e., goals and objectives that, if mastered by the children, will allow the children to communicate more effectively and appropriately in various communicative contexts). Figuring out the most reliable, valid ways to measure mastery of these functional and appropriate goals and objectives is certainly important, but we do *not* select goals and objectives for the child based on whether or not the goals and objectives themselves are easy to measure! The SCT sheet was designed to show the clinicians that there is a plan during literature-based intervention (i.e., that the session is not a haphazard catchall in which the clinician simply wings it and hopes for the best). Yet the SCT sheet also allows great flexibility in planning and implementing the session, while simultaneously illustrating just how rich a given book is in terms of the depth and complexity of language found therein.

In general, the clinician scans the text ahead of time and fills in the SCT sheet with linguistic elements from the story that he or she feels the child is likely to experience difficulty with, based on results of standardized testing, baselining, experience with prior stories, and so forth. As the child and adult facilitator proceed with the story over the course of days, the adult facilitator can check off items on the SCT sheet as the child masters them, while circling or boxing items the child appears to still be struggling with (indicating that these items will require additional scaffolding during subsequent rereadings). (Sometimes this process can take weeks if a fully developed **thematic unit**—i.e., a collection of literature and related activities such as art, drama, play, snack, or writing, that help to explore a particular topic or theme as well as enhance understanding of linguistic concepts—is being implemented.) Sometimes a child does not have difficulty with an item that was originally anticipated and targeted on the SCT sheet. If so, then that item can simply be crossed off the SCT sheet. However, even this kind of information is salient (given that prior knowledge of items or concepts can often be used to bootstrap or link with other concepts in the story or thematic unit). Other unanticipated items that the child struggles with (as exemplified by reading miscues, for example) can simply be added to the SCT sheet as the session or sessions proceed. In this manner, the SCT sheet functions not only as a lesson plan in progress but also as an assessment and measurement tool.

What follows are (1) a sample of a blank SCT sheet (Figure 4-1), (2) an SCT sheet with suggestions for the types of linguistic elements that may be targeted under each language area (e.g., morphosyntax, semantics, pragmatics, other skills and concepts) (Figure 4-2), and (3) a sample SCT sheet completed for the story *Jim's Trumpet* (Figure 4-3).

In my experience, using the SCT sheet greatly enhances the ability of beginning clinicians (and seasoned SLPs who are making the transition to literature-based intervention) to identify the elements of the story that they want to focus on with the LLD

SKILLS AND CONCEPTS TO TARGET (SCT) SHEET

Title:

Phonology (phonemes, phonemic awareness, alphabetic principle, sound-letter correspondences, rhyming, sound blending, segmentation, syllabification)

Morphosyntax (word formation, word order, grammar, sentence length/complexity)

Semantics (word meanings, word relationships, vocabulary, concept formation)

Pragmatics (using language effectively when discussing story or text during group interaction; classroom discourse; listener or speaker roles)

Other skills or concepts (thematic unit)

Figure 4-1 Skill and Concepts to Target (SCT) Sheet.

Phonology (phonemes, phonemic awareness, alphabetic principle, sound-letter correspondence, rhyming, sound blending, segmentation, syllabification)

Morphosyntax (word formation, word order, grammar, sentence length/complexity)

- Plurals
- Possessives
- Third-person singular
- Present progressive (*ing*)
- Regular past tense (*ed*)
- Irregular past tense
- Future tense
- Copula
- Auxiliary
- Negation
- Interrogatives
- Parts of speech (noun, verb, adjective, adverb, article, preposition, pronoun, conjunctions)
- Compound words
- Contractions
- Punctuation (comma, question mark, period, exclamation point, apostrophe, colon, semicolon, parentheses, hyphen)
- Simple active affirmative declarative sentence
- Passive sentence
- Compound sentence
- Complex sentence (relative clauses, subordinate clauses)
- Hierarchy (sounds and letters, syllables, words, phrases, clauses, sentences, paragraphs, chapters)

Semantics (word meanings, word relationships, vocabulary, concept formation)

- New or interesting vocabulary
- Content aspects of story or expository text (characters, personality traits, motives, how events or people are related, historical perspective)
- Synonyms
- Antonyms
- Homonyms, homophones, homographs
- Abstract or figurative language (metaphors, similes, idioms, analogies)
- Poetry, imagery

Pragmatics (using language effectively when discussing story or text during classroom interactions; classroom discourse; listener or speaker roles)

- Speech acts (labeling, requesting, repeating, answering, calling, greeting, protesting, practicing)
- Turn taking (taking a turn to speak, relinquishing turn, inviting others into conversation)
- Topic initiation, switching, maintenance
- Message repair, conciseness, brevity, efficiency, providing sufficient information to the listener, avoiding rambling, providing clarification
- Eye contact, body language, proxemics
- Prosody (rate, rhythm, intonation, inflection)
- Classroom discourse (when to talk and when not to, how to get attention such as raising hand, reading teacher's nonverbal cues, proxemics, body language, prosody such as appropriate loudness level when talking in class, what to do when you don't understand directions, how to ask for help)

Other skills and concepts to target (thematic unit)

- Thematic art, drama, games, play, snack, field trips, and any other associated activities that help explore the themes, topics, and content of the story or expository text

Figure 4-2 Suggestions for SCT Sheet.

Continued

- Concepts or themes related to the story that may not be explicitly stated in the book yet are pertinent and relevant to the topics therein
- Nonfiction or expository topics and activities related to the fictional story language

---

Figure 4-2 cont'd

child. The SCT sheet also helps clinicians feel that the literature-based sessions they are implementing are not so haphazard and random. I have often had clinicians observe my sessions and express a certain degree of amazement that I seem to know exactly what to say to the child and when to say it. In truth, much planning goes into the sessions, and when I show them my own fully completed and scripted SCT sheets, they often seem relieved when they realize that I have given a great deal of attention to the specific linguistic elements of the story I wish to scaffold and parse for the child. Yet despite having a relatively scripted and formalized plan, when I am confronted with an impromptu error on the part of the child (e.g., in the form of an oral-reading miscue or an inability to answer a constituent question), I can still easily switch tactics and deal with the child's comprehension difficulty as it occurs during the session. The SCT sheet provides a necessary degree of structure during literature-based intervention. However, it is the adult facilitator's ability to understand and utilize various scaffolding techniques, as well as to monitor the child's emerging reconstruction of meaning, that provides the necessary degree of flexibility needed to meet the child's ongoing needs during the session. It is this combination of *planning and structure* intermingled with a healthy dose of *monitoring and flexibility* that is key to effective holistic intervention with LLD children.

As a final note of encouragement, personal experience suggests that familiarity and practice with the methodology of literature-based intervention breeds competency. Clinicians using the forms and protocols become more proficient at the strategies and techniques very quickly. There is a tendency initially to mine the surface or shallower aspects of the story only, and that is perfectly acceptable. With practice and experience, clinicians quickly discover the wonderful richness and depth of children's literature and are utterly amazed at how much language

mileage they can get from just one short storybook or piece of text (*Jim's Trumpet* is a perfect example; I have often spent a very fruitful 2 to 3 weeks building a thematic unit with this story, exploring the linguistic elements, topics, and themes delineated on the SCT sheet shown in Figure 4-3). Interestingly, I have had other clinicians do an SCT sheet for this same story, and although there was always some appreciable overlap in our content, they have always managed to find themes and concepts to explore that I missed. That again is one of the beauties of this type of intervention—you never run out of language to explore with your students when you use authentic literature as your context and stimulus. The books do the work for you.

Building Thematic Units

There are several choices for how to build a thematic unit:

1. Start with a *fictional* story (e.g., *Jim's Trumpet*) and then choose *expository* or *nonfiction* texts (e.g., books about musical instruments, neighborhoods, cities, or suburbs) to expand and build on the themes that occur naturally as part of the story.
2. Start with an expository book or theme and then choose one or more fictional stories that *complement* the expository themes.
3. Go to the language arts curriculum for the child's grade level and scan textbooks and other expository materials (particularly science, social studies, or geography books). Then select fictional and expository books for intervention that complement themes from the language arts curriculum. For instance, one year, all my third-grade students were covering earth science and geology in the first few chapters of their science books (e.g., volcanoes, earthquakes, and weather-related phenomena such as

Title: *Jim's Trumpet*

Phonology (phonemes, phonemic awareness, alphabetic principle, sound-letter correspondences, rhyming, sound blending, segmentation, syllabification)

- Let's go through the book and identify words that start with consonant blends. Remember that consonant blends are two or more consonants together (*pl*ayed, *tr*umpet, *sl*eeping, *fr*iend, *st*op, *sl*eep, *pl*ease, *cl*apped)
- Is there any word on this page that starts with two consonants, but only makes one sound: the *r* sound? (*wr*ong)
- What about this word (*ch*eered)? It has two consonants at the beginning, but what sound does it tell your mouth to make? (*ch* sound)
- Here are some two–syllable words (*eating, laughing, jumping, dancing*). Can you show me how to break them into two syllables by clapping your hands for each syllable?

Morphosyntax (word formation, word order, grammar sentence length/complexity)

- Possessive (Jim*'s* trumpet, little people*'s* friend; his sister*'s* place)
- Irregular past (*sat; were*)
- Regular past (play*ed*; cheer*ed*; clapp*ed*)
- Present progressive (eat*ing*, laugh*ing*, jump*ing*, danc*ing*, sleep*ing*)
- Contractions (*can't, I'll, didn't, isn't, it's, don't*)
- Punctuation (period, exclamation point, quotation marks, comma)
- Prepositional phrases (*on* the fire escape, *to* another part of town, *at* his sister's place)

Semantics (word meanings, word relationships, vocabulary, concept formation)

- What is *soft* music vs. *eating* music and *dancing* music? (bring in cassette and play examples)
- Give examples of types of music and musical artists you like
- *Every* night (vs. *every other night, some nights, occasionally*)
- *At once* (*right away* vs. *later, soon*)
- *Fire escape* (and other *fire safety equipment* and rules in a high rise building, school)

Pragmatics (using language effectively when discussing story or text during group interaction; classroom discourse; listener or speaker roles)

- Turn taking
- Topic maintenance
- Eye contact
- Explore Jim's *body language* after he gets the news from the neighbors that he can't play his trumpet in his building anymore (i.e., head down, shoulders slumped). How does our body language reflect our feelings and moods? (Contrast with Jim's facial expression/body language after the "big people" invite him back to the building.)

Other skills or concepts (thematic unit)

- Nonfiction thematic unit on various *musical instruments*: e.g., trumpet and other wind instruments, string instruments, percussion. Discuss *orchestras, bands, careers* in music. Take field trip to symphony; have guest musician visit and perform short concert.
- What makes a *good neighbor?* What have you done to be a good neighbor (water plants, walk the dog, take in newspaper while neighbor is on vacation)?
- What makes someone a *bad neighbor?* (making too much noise, littering, parking in their parking space, letting your dog bark)? How do we resolve problems and conflicts with neighbors?
- *City living* (Jim's building) vs. living in the *suburbs* (Jim's sister's house). Where do you live? Do you like living in the city vs. the suburbs? What are the advantages/disadvantages of living in each?

Figure 4-3 Sample SCT Sheet for *Jim's Trumpet*.

tornadoes and hurricanes). I was able to find a historical fiction book about Pompeii and Mount Vesuvius. This book explored the theme of volcanoes in a very meaningful and interesting way (by discussing not only the scientific aspects of volcanoes but also what happened on a human and personal level to the people who lived in Pompeii when the volcano erupted). The book also introduced other exciting concepts related to the fields of archeology, anthropology, and history, providing even further opportunities to build and enhance the overall instructional content of the thematic unit. This book and thematic unit also provided ample opportunity for the children to gain experience using various reference and resource materials such as a globe, maps, atlases, encyclopedias, dictionaries, and other nonfiction books to locate information relevant to the topics being explored.

The creative part of the thematic unit involves planning the various art, drama, play, snack, game, writing, and any other activities designed to enhance, complement, or expand the themes of the story. Some of us are more naturally artistic, but one does not have to be a Matisse or a Picasso to plan enjoyable and meaningful thematic art activities for students. It is always wise to preserve a portfolio of thematic art activities with a sample of each finished piece (along with directions and a list of needed materials for each project). That way, you will have the art activity on file the next time you need it; remember that you will likely be using the same stories, themes, and activities over and over with different clients, groups, and classrooms over the years (with modifications, of course). I know some clinicians who keep their art, lists of thematic activities, and other literature-based materials in accordion folders or plastic bins stored by season or holiday or general thematic category. Others prefer to keep their materials separated for each story or thematic unit. The folder or bin then houses everything related to that story, including the following:

- Samples of art, dramas, play activities, games, puppets, dolls, worksheets, or writing for that story or unit

- Sample factual, interpretation, or inference questions already generated or printed out and ready to be used
- Sample SCT sheets and any other forms needed for that story or thematic unit

Keeping these materials ready to use becomes an incredible time-saver for the clinician and generally takes the place of traditional picture cards, drill sheets, and cookbook-type therapy manuals. By the way, it is always a good idea to keep your eyes open when walking down the halls of schools to escort your students back and forth to their classrooms. Teachers often display children's artwork on the walls and bulletin boards of hallways. I have gotten many excellent ideas for thematic art projects from observing students' artwork displayed in the halls of elementary schools (e.g., an octopus made from yarn and a shark made from an envelope that I ended up using quite successfully with a story about sea creatures—I certainly would have never thought of these ideas on my own!). Public libraries, bookstores, and craft stores are also replete with reference books and materials for thematically related art and other associated projects.

A word of caution about the creation of art and thematically related activities in general: always remember that it is the discussion and interaction that takes place *during* these thematically related activities (along with any scaffolding provided by the adult facilitator) that constitutes the actual *intervention*. The intervention consists of shared opportunities between the client and the adult facilitator to parse various linguistic and cognitive entities (e.g., words, sentences, paragraphs, and even whole activities) into their constituent elements, and to then reconstruct and reintegrate those components into meaningful wholes in functional contexts. The thematic activities provide the context for the interaction and intervention and often serve as the stimulus, the purpose for communication, and the natural consequence (positive or negative) of any communicative attempts as well. For instance, Box 4-2 contains a transcript of an interaction that took place during a thematic art activity involving the yarn octopus previously mentioned. The interaction involved the SLP (author) and three children from a self-contained severely language-disordered special-education class. The thematic art activity provided the opportunity to review new vocabulary and grammar, as well as opportunities

Box 4-2 Sample Interaction During Thematic Art Activity

Students. K, B, and J (three African American students enrolled in self-contained special-education classroom for severely language-disordered students; suburban elementary school; low socioeconomic status)

C: OK, since we have been reading about the greedy gray octopus, we are going to make an octopus of our own, out of yarn! Would you like to see what the octopus is going to look like when we are finished?

(K, B, and J nod affirmatively.)

C: See, his head is made out of a Styrofoam ball, and then I used *yarn* to make his body. We are going to cover his head with the yarn first and tie it tightly with a string underneath the head, so the rest of the yarn can hang free. Then, we will use all this yarn hanging down to make his legs. Who can remember how many legs an octopus has?

J: Eight legs!

C: That's correct J! And does anyone remember what we *call* the legs on an octopus?

(No response from any of the children.)

C: No one can remember what we call the legs? It's a new word that we learned last time. We read about it in the other book. The one we checked out from the library. K, could you hand me that book about sea creatures (pointing to the book on the side table). Maybe we need to review that information.

K: (Hands book to the clinician.)

C: K, can you turn the pages to the part about *octopi*? Remember, that is the *plural* of octopus; it means more than one octopus.

K: (Complies by turning to the appropriate pages, using pictures to guide him.)

C: K, do you remember what this page said about octopi—what they call the legs?

K: Some word that started with a *t*?

C: That's right, the word starts with a *t*. And here is the word (pointing to the caption under the picture of the octopus). Can you read that word?

K: Ten-ten . . . (struggles to decode the word, then trails off).

C: You got the first syllable right! Let me write it on our board. (Clinician writes the word on a dry-erase board, then draws lines to segment the word into syllables.)

Ten/ta/cles

Let's see if we can read it now that we've broken the word into syllables. Let's all read it together. Ten/ta/cles.

(All children are able to read the word once it has been segmented into syllables.)

See, it is often easier to read a long word once you break it into smaller parts. Remember to use that strategy guys, when you come across a long word. Break it into syllables! You almost always can read the syllables.

[The clinician chose the *syllabification* scaffolding strategy in this instance because the word was essentially encountered in *isolation* (i.e., in a caption under a picture, without much other textual support) and, more importantly, because semantic or meaning-based scaffolding (i.e., "Who can remember what we call the legs?") had already failed to activate the lexical item for the readers.]

C: Yes, *tentacles!* The legs of the octopus are called *tentacles!* So, you told me the octopus has eight legs, or eight *tentacles.* (Notice clinician making use of *repeating, paraphrasing,* and other CRS strategies—more discussion of CRS in next section.) So, how are we going to make eight tentacles on our yarn octopus? We have a lot of yarn here to work with!

B: We could tie some of these yarns together so there's only eight of 'em.

C: You're right B! We could tie some of the *strands of yarn* together so that we make eight separate clumps that look like legs. But what could we use to tie the strands of yarn together?

B: Well, we gots some yarn left over (pointing to the ball of yarn next to the clinician).

C: That's true, we do *have* some yarn left over, and we could cut some of it into strips to tie clumps of yarn together to make legs. But I can think of another way. Look at J's hair (J is the only female student in the group).

(All students look at J's hair.)

C: J, can you tell us what kind of hairstyle you have?

J: Braids!

C: Yes you do! You have really pretty braids in your hair! Do you know how to braid hair?

J: I do! My Momma did my braids, but I know how too!

C: I'm really glad to hear that because I think *braiding* the yarn to make eight separate legs would be a really neat way to do it! What do you all think?

C, Clinician; *CRS,* communicative reading strategies.

Continued

Box 4-2 Sample Interaction During Thematic Art Activity—cont'd

(J nods excitedly, but K and B look dubious.)

K: I don't know how to braid.

J: That's OK. I can teach you!

C: What a great idea! J, you can give us a demonstration of how to braid using the yarn hanging from your octopus head. And be sure to *explain* the steps in the procedure as you do it. You're going to give us *directions* on how to braid.
   Remember we talked about how to give good directions.

C, Clinician.

for problem solving, verbal turn taking, topic initiation and maintenance, requesting and giving information, and phonological awareness activities.

Scaffolding During Oral Reading Using Communicative Reading Strategies

Definition

Up to this point I have used the term *scaffolding* with the assumption that the reader has a basic understanding of the term. Now I will go into more detail. What do we mean by this term? And what does scaffolding have to do with what we do during literature-based intervention?

The metaphor for scaffolding comes from the scaffold that we often see erected temporarily around buildings that are being constructed or renovated. This scaffolding (which in the real world may be made of metal or wood and may involve various other structures such as crossbeams or catwalks) is designed to provide *temporary* support for the workers (and possibly the emerging structure itself) during the construction or renovation. But as the new or remodeled structure emerges and gains strength, pieces of the scaffolding are gradually removed. Eventually, as the building proceeds and the scaffolding is removed, the structure is capable of standing alone. However, if the scaffolding is too weak initially or is removed too soon, the building will be in danger of losing its structural integrity and may collapse. Likewise, when working with LLD children, the adult facilitator provides scaffolding in forms such as assistance, cues, or modeling to help the child perform at a level he or she would not otherwise be capable of performing

without assistance. As the child gradually gains strength (like the emerging building) or mastery over the task, the adult facilitator gradually withdraws or removes the scaffolding, so that the child is eventually performing the task independently.

What Are Communicative Reading Strategies?

Communicative reading strategies (CRS) (Norris, 1988, 1989, 1991) consist of a variety of scaffolding principles and techniques that have been used successfully to improve both oral and written language deficits in language-disordered children (Badon, 1993; DeKemel, 1998; Ezell, 1995; Hernandez, 1989).

CRS is a **communication-based approach** to reading, designed to facilitate the reader's ability to construct multiple levels of meaning representation from the text. Intervention with CRS involves conducting the reading event as a **meaning-making process,** and all cueing systems (e.g., visual, auditory, graphophonemic, picture, context, prior knowledge, previously read information) are utilized to help the reader process the meaning of the text and the underlying information (Norris & Hoffman, 1993). CRS takes the form of **scaffolded dialogue** between the LLD child and the adult facilitator, with the adult facilitator providing more or less assistance (scaffolding) as needed to help the reader decipher the language and reconstruct the intended meaning of the text. When using CRS, one should pay particular attention to the reader's fluency and word recognition, because oral-reading miscues frequently provide clues to the reader's decoding and comprehension difficulties (see Chapter 2), and scaffolding strategies are adjusted accordingly. When the text is difficult for the child (as evidenced by multiple reading miscues or struggle behaviors), the adult facilitator may provide more scaffolding (particularly in the form of parsing a sentence, phrase, or word into its constituent parts) to help the child make sense of the content, form, or surface features of the text. When the text is less difficult, the adult facilitator may assist the child in making more abstract interpretations, inferences, and evaluations about the text (Norris & Hoffman, 1993). Over time, children generally require less and less scaffolding as they become more independent, strategic readers, capable of constructing meaning at multiple levels of representation.

Although practitioners using CRS generally employ a variety of scaffolding techniques, perhaps one of the most important features involves an adaptation of what has been referred to in the literature as the **method of repeated readings** (Dowhower, 1997; LaBerge & Samuels, 1974; Samuels, 1976). Dowhower (1997) notes that the method of repeated readings usually involves having the student "reread a short, meaningful passage several times until a satisfactory level of fluency is reached." This method was originally based on the **automaticity theory** (LaBerge & Samuels, 1974; Samuels, 1976), which suggests that fluent readers are those who decode text automatically, thus leaving their attention free for comprehension. Dowhower (1997) notes that the method of repeated readings has had a significant impact on educational practice for the last 2 decades and has been adapted and used successfully by a variety of reading practitioners, including those who subscribe to holistic-interactive philosophy, as well as skills-based reading methods. Studies have shown the method of repeated readings to be particularly beneficial to poor readers, resulting not only in increased fluency but in improved motivation and greater self-confidence as well (Dowhower, 1997).

The method of repeated readings has been adapted for use in CRS in the following manner. First, rather than reading an entire story in one sitting, the child reads *only a few pages* of a story at a time. As the child prepares to read the first few pages of text, scaffolding is used to facilitate the student's activation of relevant background knowledge, ability to utilize picture and contextual cues (e.g., by looking at the title, cover page, and pictures), and ability to make predictions about the content of the story. As the child reads, *miscues are addressed as they occur*, and scaffolding strategies to assist comprehension are employed accordingly.

On subsequent occasions, the student may be asked to verbally summarize what has already happened in the story (sometimes with the help of a graphic organizer such as a story map [described later in the chapter] or flow chart) and to reread previously read pages of the story before proceeding on to new pages. Careful attention is again paid to any remaining miscues when the student rereads a portion of the text, and additional scaffolding is provided accordingly. Students may exhibit poor fluency and multiple miscues during their first reading of a piece of text, but with each successive reading, they generally produce fewer miscues, and the rate, phrasing, and fluency often improve as well. These improvements may be attributed to a combination of scaffolding and repeated exposure to the same piece of text, such that decoding and processing difficulties are gradually overcome. In other words, the focus when using CRS and the method of repeated readings is *not* on reading the story as quickly as possible, but rather on building comprehension and fluency as the child reads and rereads meaningful and interesting material in context. In addition, by breaking down a longer story into manageable parts, the child has the opportunity to master one part of the story before going on to the next, resulting in a type of cumulative **constructive comprehension**. Mastering each part of the story successively also allows the child to experience frequent successes while reading. This may be particularly helpful with LLD or poor readers for whom the reading event has seldom been a successful or enjoyable experience. Students may gain much needed confidence and motivation as a result.

Other advantages to using CRS include the following: (1) the techniques may be used with individuals or small groups of children and may even be modified for use in classroom settings when implemented as part of a collaborative language lesson on the part of the SLP and classroom teacher; (2) the adult facilitator is provided with a flexible set of strategies for addressing the reader's decoding and comprehension difficulties while the child is actually reading the text; (3) unlike many phonics- and skills-based reading remediation programs, CRS focuses on helping the child become a balanced reader, capable of using multiple strategies for decoding and comprehending text; and (4) it provides a way to help the reader work on constructing progressively more abstract interpretations and inferences about the text, as opposed to focusing solely on extraction of literal, explicit information. Most importantly, with its focus on simultaneous bottom-up and top-down processing, CRS is consistent with the constructionist-connectionist model of cognition discussed in Chapter 1.

For these reasons, CRS has great potential as a remediation technique for LLD children who exhibit a variety of problems with decoding, comprehension, and inferential processing during the reading of narrative and expository texts. (Box 4-3 lists CRS techniques with specific examples.)

Box 4-3 Communicative Reading Strategies

Preparatory Sets

Assist the reader in activating appropriate background knowledge
Link new information to previously stated ideas in the story
Help reader learn to expect meaning when reading
Help reader remain focused on the theme or topic of the passage
Direct reader to more abstract interpretations of language in story
Can prep set any linguistic unit of text (word, phrase, sentence, paragraph)

Examples: Text says, "Effy was hot, so she turned on a fan. The fan blew a candle. The flame flipped into a pan. Effy huffed and puffed at the flame to snuff out the fire. But that made the flame flare higher and higher!"
Prep set: "Find out who was hot." (labels)
    "Tell us what Effy is doing." (actions)
    "Tell us how Effy feels." (interpretations)
    "Find out if blowing on the fire worked." (inferences)
    "Which words have the /f/ sound in the beginning/middle/ending?" (metalanguage)

Constituent Questions

Are similar to prep sets (with focus on alerting child to information that is needed) but require that child reverse interrogative syntactic forms as opposed to responding to more direct form of prep set

Example: "What caused the fire to flip into a pan?"

Acknowledgment

Provides feedback to reader by confirming what has been read and understood
Treats reading as natural communicative act in which speakers and listeners take turns and attempt to communicate meaningful information

Example: Text says, "Effy was hot so she turned on a fan."
Acknowledgment: "Oh, it must be a hot summer day."

Expansion

Rewords text information into grammatically more complete or complex sentence
Uses more complete or complex sentences; generally include relational terms, such as conjunctions (e. g., *because, so, when*), verb tense markers (e. g., *will, did, should*), adjectives, adverbs, or subordinate clauses

Example: Text says, "The fan blew a candle."
Expansion: "The fan blew the flame away from the candle."

Expatiation

Consists of elaborations on idea or concept to establish greater meaning, to clarify unfamiliar vocabulary or concepts, to explain metaphor or other figurative language, or to model inferences and interpretations

Example: Text says, "But that made the flame flare higher and higher!"
Expatiation: "Blowing on the flame didn't snuff out the fire. It did the opposite. It made the flame suddenly flare or get bigger."

Developed by Janet Norris, Ph.D., CCC-SLP, Department of Communication Sciences and Disorders, Louisiana State University, Baton Rouge, LA.

Box 4-3 Communicative Reading Strategies—cont'd

Association

Establishes links between new information read and ideas that have been stated in previous episodes, pages, paragraphs or sentences

Helps reader understand that meaning crosses boundaries of sentences, paragraphs, and pages (i.e., cohesion)

Example: Text says, "The fan blew a candle."
Association: Clinician reviews previous page and makes association such as "Effy turned on a fan to cool herself, but that caused a new problem. It caused . . ." (pointing to new text).

Generalization

Links events, morals, or states in story to similar situations in other contexts, such as reader's own experiences or community, national, or world events

Example: Text says, "But that made the flame flare higher and higher!"
Generalization: "That's what we learned in fire safety. Don't run because air makes a fire flare."

Parsing

Chunks complex sentences into smaller units to aid processing of ideational relationships within sentences
Helps reader to see how sentence is made up of smaller constituents and semantic units

Example: Text says, "Effy huffed and puffed at the flame to snuff out the fire."
Parsing: "Find out how Effy tried to put out the fire." (pointing to the word *flame*); "She was trying to do this." (pointing to *snuff out the fire*)

Semantic Cue

Assists in retrieving or recognizing a word that is miscued or difficult to decode
Gives synonyms, definitions, or related words to help establish correct network of information
May model word in context if word is not in the child's lexicon

Example: If child miscues on word *snuff.*
Semantic cue: "This word means to put out a candle; to put out a flame quickly."

Fluent Reading

Is used to model how elements of sentence work together to communicate meaning
Is used when reader struggles with text and other scaffolding strategies alone are not successful in helping reader to construct meaning
Directs reader to look at written words while facilitator reads
Simultaneously lets reader see and hear how sentence or phrase functions as a whole

Example: If child reads, "The fan blew a cand-, candy, canlee."
Fluent Reading: Clinician models fluent reading of sentence, "The fan blew a candle," followed by expatiation or other scaffolding strategy, to help child associate words with meaning.

Paraphrase

Is used to reword text after it is read
May reduce difficulty of vocabulary or concept
May define unfamiliar words through descriptions or use of synonyms
Can reword complex sentences in shorter, simpler sentences
Can model interpretations, inferences, or other cues to more abstract meaning

Example: Text says, "But that made the flame flare higher and higher!"
Paraphrase: "Blowing on the fire caused the flame to get bigger and taller."

Continued

Box 4-3 Communicative Reading Strategies—cont'd

Summarization

Can be oral retelling or summary of previously read information

Can include rereading parts of passages to integrate ideas

Examples: "Can you explain to us what has happened so far in the story?"
"Can you tell us what happened on this page?"
"Can you read that paragraph again for us?"

Graphic Organizers

Are visual representations of information consisting of key words or concepts in visual array

Allow for metalinguistic analysis of story grammar constituents (e.g., characters, setting, initiating event, plans, attempts, resolutions, moral) and understanding of how author constructs story for reader

Allow topic or concepts to be held in focus long enough to be compared and placed in relationship with new and old information

Can be reviewed for recall

Help child learn how to retell or summarize a story

Examples: flow charts, diagrams, semantic webs, story maps, time lines

Turn Assistance

Has clinician, on completing turn in dialogue about story, supply form of turn assistance to cue child to take next turn

Forms of turn assistance include the following:

Binary Choice

Example: "Did the flame get bigger or smaller?"

Cloze Procedure

Examples: "Effy turned on a . . . (fan) because she was too . . . (hot)."
"It surprised her when the flame . . . (flipped into a pan)."

Cloze Procedure With Pointing and Gestures

Example: "When she was hot, Effy turned . . ." (gesturing as if turning a knob).
"That fan was too close to the . . ." (pointing to the candle).

Cloze Procedure With Phonemic Cues

Example: "Effy huffed at the /f/ . . ." (flame).
"That made the fire /f/ . . ." (flare).

Cloze Procedure With Relational Terms

Examples: "Effy was hot so . . ." (she turned on the fan).
"The flame flew into a pan after . . ." (the fan blew a candle).
"Effy tried to snuff out the fire but . . ." (it flared even higher).

Developed by Janet Norris, Ph.D., CCC-SLP, Department of Communication Sciences and Disorders, Louisiana State University, Baton Rouge, LA.

Use of Story Maps and Other Graphic Organizers During Literature-Based Intervention

A **story map** is defined as a graphic representation of all or part of the elements of a story and the relationships between them (Davis & McPherson, 1989). Most fictional stories are organized along universal **story grammars** or **story schemata**, containing elements such as characters, setting (time and place), an initiating event, a problem, a plan, actions (events or reactions), and an outcome or resolution (Stein & Glenn, 1979). Story maps may serve as idealized mental representations of story structure and provide a practical means for children to integrate literal and implicit information about characters and events into an organized whole (Beck & McKeown, 1981). Davis and McPherson (1989) note that story maps can be created in a variety of forms to meet individual needs of students including (1) **locating-information story maps,** which help the student locate or retrieve literal or factual information from the story; (2) **inferential story maps,** which help the student make inferences and draw conclusions; (3) **cause-and-effect story maps,** which help the student make connections between character motives, actions, and outcomes; and (4) **comparison** or **contrast story maps,** which help the student compare or contrast characters' traits, motives, and circumstances, as well as compare or contrast different stories. Story maps can be used (1) *before reading* to assist students in activating prior knowledge and making predictions, (2) *during reading* to chart ongoing events and help the readers stay focused, or (3) *after reading* to help students recall or reconstruct what happened in the story. Story maps may focus on a particular episode within a story or on the total structure of the story as a whole (Hoggan & Strong, 1994).

Various studies support the premise that the use of story maps and instruction about story parts does result in improved reading comprehension (Gordon and Pearson, 1983; Idol, 1987; Reutzel, 1984). Story maps can be used as an instructional strategy across the curriculum to incorporate all four of the language modalities (reading, writing, speaking, listening), encompassing a variety of grade levels and content areas. Figure 4-4 shows a sample story map format that may be used during literature-based intervention, and Figure 4-5 contains a completed sample story map for the story *Jim's Trumpet*.

Suggestions for Using a Story Map

I find that one of the best ways to use a story map is at the end of each session, as a way to summarize the events that have occurred on the pages read during that session. Sample directions from the clinician to the client before filling out each section of the story map are shown in Figure 4-6.

The child and the clinician may only fill out one or two sections of the story map per session (depending on how many pages of the story were read and covered that day). During the next session, time is always spent reviewing the parts of the story map that have already been completed. With time and with this type of consistent reviewing, the child will internalize the story map constituents, which in turn helps to improve narrative comprehension and narrative-retelling abilities.

Completion of the story map also provides a wonderful opportunity to work on writing and spelling abilities (see Chapter 6). Although the focus of the story map should be primarily on the story elements themselves, its creation still constitutes an authentic writing activity whose purpose is to convey meaning. In this case, the goal is for the child to generate a graphic organizer that results in better self-organization and recall of the essential story grammar elements and, ultimately, better narrative retelling ability.

Character Maps

Another useful graphic organizer is the character map, which facilitates the student's understanding of character traits and motives. Character maps are particularly beneficial as students move to more advanced literary analysis in upper elementary, middle, and high school (e.g., when teachers expect them to analyze and explain *why* characters act as they do in the story). I have even had success using character maps with adult LLD college students who are involved with advanced literature such as the Shakespearean dramas *Hamlet* and *MacBeth*. In terms of enhancing lexical development and the writing of paragraphs or essays, character maps are a wonderful way to help the student focus on the development of adjectives (which are often needed

Title:

Characters (who):

Setting (where, when):

Initiating Event:

Problem:

Plans or Attempts:

Consequences

Resolution:

Moral:

Figure 4-4 Story Map.

Title: *Jim's Trumpet*

Characters (who): Jim, the little people, the big people, Jim's sister

Setting (where, when): Jim's building (the fire escape), Jim's sister's house, Jim's building

Initiating event: Jim played the trumpet for the little people in his building, and they really liked his music.

Problem: But the two big people did not like Jim's trumpet music. They were bothered by the noise, and they told him to stop playing.

Plans or Attempts: Jim didn't want to stop playing his trumpet, so he went to live at his sister's house, where he could keep on playing.

Consequences: The little people and the big people in Jim's building missed the trumpet music. They couldn't sleep without it.

Resolution: So the big people went to Jim's sister's house and asked Jim to come back. They told him they liked his music after all. So Jim went back and played his music again and everyone was happy, including the big people.

Moral: We should be considerate of our neighbors' feelings. And sometimes, when there is something in our lives that we think we don't like, we end up missing it when it's gone!

Figure 4–5 Sample Story Map for *Jim's Trumpet.*

Clinician: What was the title of our story? Let's write that here next to *Title* on the story map. Where do we find the title of the story? That's right, on the cover of the book.

Clinician: The next part of the story map says *Characters*. That means the people or animals in the story. Let's list the characters we have met so far.

Clinician: The next part of the story map says *Setting*. That means, where and when did the actions in the story take place? Where are the characters at the beginning of the story? Let's list that information here. Remember, the setting can change as the story goes along, so we may have to list different settings as we read further along in the book.

Clinician: The next part of the story map says *Initiating Event*. That means, what happened at the beginning of the story that got the action started? Let's think of a sentence that summarizes the initiating event.

Clinician: The next part of the story map says *Problem*. That means, What problem did the character have that needed to be solved? Let's think of a sentence (or two) that summarizes the character's problem.

Clinician: The next part of the story map says *Plans or Attempts*. That means, What attempts did the character make to solve the problem? Let's think of a summary sentence (or two or three) to describe what the character did to solve the problem.

Clinician: The next part of the story map says *Consequences*. That means, What were the consequences or results of the character's attempts to solve the problem? Was the character successful in solving the problem? Let's write a summary sentence (or two or three) to describe the consequences.

Clinician: The next part of the story map says *Resolution*. That means the ending, or How did the story resolve itself? Did the story have a happy ending? Let's write a summary sentence or two to describe the resolution.

Clinician: The final part of the story map says *Moral*. That means, What lesson about life did we learn from the story? What lesson did the characters learn? Let's write that here.

Figure 4–6 Directions to Client for Filling in a Story Map.

to adequately describe character traits). LLD students are often very "static" in their description of characters (both their physical traits and emotional characteristics). I often let them start their character map using their relatively static descriptors and then assist them in using a thesaurus to locate synonyms to replace these static terms with more colorful, vibrant descriptors that truly capture the essence of the character. For example, a child is filling out the character map for Jack from *Jack in the Beanstalk;* if the child writes, *Bad, doesn't listen to his mother,* to describe one of Jack's personality traits, I might provide additional assistance in the form of verbal scaffolding and use of a children's thesaurus to help the child discover new lexical items such as *disobedient, willful,* and *naughty.* It is also advisable to have LLD students contrast one character's habits and traits with those of another character in the story (this type of contrastive character analysis is often the very thing that teachers of literature are looking for when grading essays). Boxes 4-4 and 4-5 show two sample character maps: one for *Jim's Trumpet* and one for the classic fairy tale *Jack and the Beanstalk.*

Measuring Other Abilities and Skills During Literature-Based Intervention

If you refer back to the SCT sheet (see Figure 4-1), you can see that multiple linguistic parameters (i.e.,

phonology, morphology, semantics, syntax, and pragmatics) are addressed and targeted during literature-based intervention. We have already explored how oral-reading miscue analysis, question comprehension, and narrative retelling can be used for baselining and measuring progress during intervention. But there are a variety of ways to document and assess progress in the other linguistic domains from the SCT sheet as well. Chapter 5 contains detailed information about the lexicon and vocabulary acquisition in the LLD population. However, given that we are focusing on forms and protocols for assessment and documenting treatment progress, it seems pertinent to include the **vocabulary**

Box 4-4 Sample Character Map for *Jim's Trumpet*

Character: Jim
Age and Gender: Young boy, probably age 10 or 11 years
Where He Lives: Apartment building; in the city
Lifestyle: Likes to play the trumpet; has a lot of friends (the little people)
Personality: Friendly, passionate (about his trumpet playing), talented

Character: The Big People
Age and Gender: Grown-ups, probably husband and wife
Where They Live: Apartment building; in the city
Lifestyle: Probably work during the day
Personality: Like quiet; need their sleep at night

Box 4-5 Sample Character Map for *Jack and the Beanstalk**

Character: Jack
Age and Gender: Young boy
Where He Lives: In the country; in a cottage; with his mother
Lifestyle: Poor
Personality:
  Curious
  Bold
  Brave
  Foolish
  Greedy
  Clever
  Cunning
  Careful
  Caring (about his mother)

Character: The Giant
Age and Gender: Older man
Where He Lives: In a castle; above the clouds; with his wife
Lifestyle: Rich
Personality:
  Mean-spirited
  Greedy
  Lazy
  Slovenly
  Cruel (to his wife)
  Selfish
  Gluttonous
  Careless (falls asleep)

*A similar character map could be constructed to compare and contrast the two female characters in the book: Jack's mother and the Giant's wife.

Box 4-6 Vocabulary and New Concept Scoring System

0 = Student has no idea what word or concept means; cannot identify, describe, define, or utilize item expressively in context.

1 = Student has limited idea of what word or concept means; may be able to identify, describe, define (with prompting or cueing), but still cannot use word or concept spontaneously and expressively in context (e.g., when retelling or discussing story).

2 = Student has fully developed understanding of what word or concept means (able to identify, describe, define); beginning to be able to use expressively in limited fashion (with prompting or cueing).

3 = Student has fully developed understanding of what word or concept means; can identify, describe, define, and utilize word or concept correctly and spontaneously in context when retelling or discussing story.

and new concept scoring system (Box 4-6) in this chapter. This scoring system has proved to be useful in documenting the acquisition of novel words and concepts children encounter in fictional and expository texts. Table 4-1 shows a chart from a group of school-age LLD children over time, documenting each child's acquisition of vocabulary from the story *Ali Baba* (De La Touche, 1995) using the vocabulary and new concept scoring system.

A similar system has been devised to document the student's acquisition of grammar and morphosyntactical elements during literature-based intervention (Box 4-7). This box is followed by data from a series of consecutive sessions, illustrating how progress on morphosyntactical elements from a real story was documented for a school-age LLD student named Adam (Table 4-2).

Incorporating Expository Texts Into Thematic Units

As previously indicated, expository texts (i.e., non-fiction materials) form an essential part of any well-built thematic unit. Expository texts may be defined

Table 4-1 Sample Group Chart Using Vocabulary and New Concept Scoring System With Story *Ali Baba*

NAME/DATE	MERCHANT	BANDITS	ASTONISH	ALLAH	BAGHDAD	"NOSE IN THE AIR"
Sally						
4-1-02	1	1	1	0	0	0
4-3-02	2	1	1	1	1	1
4-7-02	2	2	1	1	1	1
4-9-02	3	3	2	2	2	2
Robbie						
4-1-02	1	1	2	0	0	1
4-3-02	2	1	1	1	0	1
4-7-02	2	1	2	1	1	1
4-9-02	2	2	2	1	1	1
Brett						
4-1-02	2	2	2	1	1	1
4-3-02	2	2	2	2	1	2
4-7-02	2	2	2	2	2	2
4-9-02	3	3	3	2	2	3

Source: Ali Baba, by G. De La Touche, 1995, New York: Shooting Star Press. Copyright © Grandreams Limited.
Lexical items across top.
Students' names at left.
Number in each cell is score from vocabulary and new concept scoring system, reflecting student's acquisition or mastery of each lexical item over time (across sessions).

Box 4-7 Grammar and Morphosyntax Scoring System

0 = Student has no idea what morphosyntactic element means or how it is used (i.e., cannot explain what structural element means or how it functions; may not use correctly in either spoken or written mode).

1 = Student has some idea of what morphosyntactic element means and how it is used (perhaps can explain in limited fashion formal grammar rule; may be able to perform limited receptive tasks such as fill in blank or multiple choice worksheet type of activities involving that morphosyntactic rule or structure); still may not use structure or rule correctly (expressively) in either spoken or written mode.

2 = Student has more fully developed sense of what morphosyntactic structure means and how it is used (getting better at explaining the formal grammar rule); structure may be used correctly (but perhaps still inconsistently) in verbal or written mode.

3 = Student has fully developed sense of what morphosyntactic structure means and how it is used (can explain formal grammar rule); structure is used correctly and consistently in both verbal and written mode.

as *informational texts* (Slater, 1988). According to Slater, the purpose of an expository text is to "present and explain theories, predictions, persons, facts, dates, specifications, generalizations, limitations, and conclusions to the reader." Expository text can sometimes be very barren in form; that is, the author may present the expository information without taking into account the potential reader's needs or degree of background knowledge (Anderson, 1985). Therefore, the reader of the expository text must (as with narrative text) synthesize and analyze information, make interpretations and inferences, and otherwise engage in constructive comprehension in order to grasp the intended meaning of the text.

Fortunately, authors of expository text do not completely leave their readers without guidance; good expository text is often very directive and contains a variety of very predictable organizational structures. Expository authors often provide explicit **metadiscourse** in the form of introductions, headings and subheadings, transitions, and summaries to assist the reader in comprehending the main and supporting ideas (Slater, 1988). Armed with a clear understanding of the purpose and organizational structure of expository text, the adult facilitator will be prepared to provide the LLD child with much-needed scaffolding to assist in constructive comprehension and recall.

As with the narrative genre, there is a plethora of research regarding the structure of expository text,

Table 4-2 Sample Chart Using Grammar and Morphosyntax Scoring System With Story *Ali Baba**

Student: Adam

COMPLEX VERB CONSTRUCTIONS Date *(Score)*	COMPARATIVES AND SUPERLATIVES Date *(Score)*	ADVERBS Date *(Score)*
"His wife despair*ed* of *their ever being* rich."	"Their leader was the cruelest of them all."	Cautious*ly*
4-1-02 *(0)*	4-1-02 *(0)*	4-1-02 *(0)*
4-3-02 *(1)*	4-3-02 *(0)*	4-3-02 *(1)*
4-8-02 *(1)*	4-8-02 *(1)*	4-8-02 *(1)*
4-10-02 *(1)*	4-10-02 *(2)*	4-10-02 *(2)*
". . .far more than Ali Baba *had ever seen*."	"We will be even wealth*ier* than we are now!"	"He gen*tly* carried his brother's body. . ."
4-1-02 *(1)*	4-1-02 *(0)*	4-1-02 *(1)*
4-3-02 *(1)*	4-3-02 *(1)*	4-3-02 *(2)*
4-8-02 *(2)*	4-8-02 *(1)*	4-8-02 *(2)*
4-10-02 *(3)*	4-10-02 *(2)*	4-10-02 *(3)*

Source: Ali Baba, by G. De La Touche, 1995, New York: Shooting Star Press. Copyright © Grandreams Limited.
Number in parentheses indicates score using grammar and morphosyntax scoring system.

the development of the ability to comprehend expository text, and the use of expository text in the elementary and secondary school curriculum. First, it appears that readers from fourth grade through college show increasing ability to use main ideas and/or the structure of expository text to facilitate recall and comprehension (Slater, 1988). According to Slater, numerous studies conducted with readers in elementary school, middle school, high school, and college have consistently shown that readers' ability to use text structure and main ideas for comprehension is a skill that increases with age (i.e., it reflects a developmental trend). Baker and Brown (1984) also concluded that the ability to fully capitalize on expository text structure and main ideas for comprehension purposes is apparently a late-developing skill (i.e., fourth grade and above).

Slater (1988) summarized research findings in the area of expository text structure as follows:

1. Readers from fourth grade through college increasingly develop their ability to use expository text structure and/or main ideas to facilitate comprehension and recall.
2. Readers who can identify and use text structure and main ideas remember more of what they read than do readers who cannot or do not use text structure and main ideas.
3. Main ideas are retained better than low-level ideas.
4. Readers can be taught to identify expository text structure and main ideas.
5. Training in the use of text structure and main ideas improves reading comprehension.

6. Failure to use expository text structure and main ideas has a more negative impact when the topic of the material is unfamiliar than when it is familiar (i.e., familiarity with the topic or degree of the reader's background knowledge makes a difference).

Slater (1988) also points out that it is essential that writers incorporate the metadiscourse cues previously mentioned (e.g., introductions, headings, subheadings, transitions) into their written expositions to facilitate readers' comprehension. Because young children (in grades below fourth grade) and LLD students may be expected to possess limited knowledge of expository text structure and metadiscourse cues, these areas provide logical points for scaffolding and teachable moments while these children are engaged in authentic writing activities with the adult facilitator.

Given that the purposes of reading expository text and the organizational structure of the text are different from those of the narrative genre, different graphic organizers are needed as well. Table 4-3 provides an example of a **fact map,** a type of graphic organizer that is very useful to create *before* having the LLD child read a piece of expository text. The purpose of the fact map is to help the child generate appropriate background knowledge before reading (again, bearing in mind that failure to identify main ideas often results in poorer comprehension and recall, especially when the topic is unfamiliar or the reader fails to activate relevant background knowledge). This is accomplished by first urging the child to engage in the **metacognitive** strategy of asking, "What do I already know about the topic?" and

Table 4-3 Sample Fact Map for Volcanoes

COLUMN A: WHAT I ALREADY KNOW	COLUMN B: WHAT I WANT TO KNOW	COLUMN C: WHAT I FOUND OUT
Some volcanoes erupt, and some do not.	What do we call scientists who study volcanoes?	(Enter in data after reading is complete.)
Hot lava comes out of volcanoes, and when the lava cools, it turns into rock.	What is lava made of and what is lava called when it is still inside the volcano?	(Enter in data after reading is complete.)
Volcanoes look like a regular mountain when they are not erupting.	What else comes out of a volcano besides lava?	(Enter in data after reading is complete.)
People live near volcanoes even though they are dangerous.	How are volcanoes formed and what makes them erupt?	(Enter in data after reading is complete.)
There are volcanoes all over the world.	How many volcanoes are there in the United States and where are they located?	(Enter in data after reading is complete.)

then listing that information in column A of the fact map. Then the clinician and child work together to identify information that the child wants to know by reading the expository text. This helps guide the LLD reader by activating a plan for reading ahead of time. By listing what he or she wants to know or learn, the LLD child generates a *purpose* for reading and will therefore be alert and watching for the information needed to answer the questions listed on the fact map while the text is read. Furthermore, part of scaffolding during oral reading of the expository text may involve going back and forth between the text and the fact map to ensure that key information is being located and processed—that the "what I want to know" answers from column B are indeed being satisfactorily addressed. It is also important to make sure that the child verifies the accuracy of the information in the "what I already know" statements from column A of the fact map while the expository text is being read. (This is a wonderful opportunity to point out to the child that many times we *think* we know something, only to discover that the information is false or inaccurate when we check it against formal resource materials).

After the completion of the reading and discussion of the expository text, the actual answers to the questions from column B (plus any other new and vital information that was learned while reading) are recorded in column C of the fact map. Discussing and adding information to the fact map before, during, and after completion of the reading helps the child identify main ideas, thus facilitating comprehension and recall. The fact map itself may also be used as a scaffold for any type of formal writing, test taking, or verbal summary activity (e.g., expository retelling, a study guide for a text or quiz, a paragraph or essay-writing exercise, a chapter summary) that takes place after the reading.

There are many ways to measure progress in the realm of expository discourse. Oral-miscue analysis along with measuring the accuracy of responses to factual, interpretation, and inference questions as discussed in previous chapters is certainly a valid and reliable method. Given that children are often asked to verbally summarize information they have read in their expository textbooks (e.g., a chapter or section in their science or social studies book), an **expository retelling rating scale** seems appropriate as well. Figure 4-7 shows an example

of an expository retelling rating scale that may be used to assess the child's ability to summarize factual information while adhering to essential expository organizational structure.

Final Comments on Measuring Treatment Progress

It is important to note that the data collection and record-keeping suggestions listed earlier are just suggestions. Different SLPs, teachers, and related service providers may devise documentation and record-keeping procedures far superior to anything I have suggested in this text, but I hope that the various charts and scoring systems provided here will at least give the service provider preliminary tools for documenting students' progress and the efficacy of treatment when using literature-based intervention. As previously stated, the fear of *not* being able to accurately, reliably, and efficiently document progress when using literature-based intervention is often *the* major obstacle clinicians cite in refusing to try this therapeutic paradigm in the first place. But in reality there is little to fear. The procedures are not carved in stone—it is almost a certainty that we will continue to refine our procedures for measuring and documenting the progress of treatment in the future. This has been (and always will be) a challenge for our discipline. We will always need to develop measurement tools that are descriptive and accurate, flexible and efficient, and yet not overly time-consuming to use. That is a tall order to fill, and we must continue to work collaboratively to achieve it.

Sample Individual Education Plan Objectives

When I present instructional content about literature-based intervention at professional conferences for teachers, SLPs, and related service providers, I am always asked to provide concrete behavioral objectives that can be used for individualized education plans (IEPs). In this instance, I am happy to oblige! Box 4-8 shows a series of IEP objectives that correlate with information provided in this chapter and others. In the appendixes of this book, I provide a sample lesson plan that presents the same information in a slightly altered format for those

---

Client Name: _____   Date: _____

Title of Expository Text: _____   Examiner: _____

SCORING SYSTEM

0 = No evidence
1 = Partial evidence
2 = Complete evidence

OBLIGATORY FEATURES (score 0, 1, or 2 for each item)

1. Includes all main (superordinate) ideas   _____
2. Includes sufficient supporting (subordinate) details.   _____
3. Exhibits text organization such as descriptive (attributes), comparative-contrastive, causative (antecedent-consequence; problem-solution), or collective (sequence or enumeration)   _____
4. Summarizes or paraphrases rather than lists details   _____
5. Is cohesive (uses connectives and other linguistic devices so that retelling flows smoothly)   _____
                                                                          Subtotal _____

OPTIONAL FEATURES

Add one point for each of the following if present:

1. Interprets or infers beyond text to world or background knowledge or own life   _____
2. Asks or suggests additional information not encountered in text that is relevant or related in content or meaning to text   _____
3. Gives relevant opinions about text content and justifies opinions   _____
                                                                          Subtotal _____

Subtract one point for each of the following if present:

1. Adds irrelevant or extraneous information not in original text   _____
2. Gives incorrect information or details   _____

                                                                          TOTAL _____

Modified from "Richness of retelling scale," B. Moss, 1997, *Reading Research and Instruction, 37(1),* 1–13 and P. A. Irwin & J. N. Mitchell. "A procedure for assessing the richness of retellings," 1983, *Journal of Reading, 26,* 394–395.

Figure 4–7 Expository Retelling Scale.

who may wish to accompany the behavioral objectives with teaching strategies, a list of media and materials, and a section for listing evaluation and the carryover of activities for the next session.

Summary

In this chapter we have covered procedures for beginning therapy after obtaining initial baseline data, how to select books at the student's instructional reading level, how to build thematic units, and a variety of methods for measuring and documenting the progress of treatment during literature-based intervention. I also explored actual scaffolding pro-

cedures to be used during the interactive dialogue that takes place during oral reading (i.e., communicative reading strategies) and examined a sample transcript of an interaction between a clinician and a group of LLD students during a thematic art activity. In essence, I provided an organizational structure for planning and implementing literature-based intervention to counter the critics who often argue that this type of intervention is too disorganized, or too loosely structured, thus making it difficult or impossible to write clear behavioral goals and objectives for the client, much less document the progress of treatment. I hope that forms such as the SCT sheet, the vocabulary and new concept scoring system, and

Box 4-8 Sample Individualized Education Plan Objectives for Literature-Based Intervention

1. Student will retell narratives in correct sequence and detail, adhering to **story grammar elements** (i.e., adequate description of *characters, setting, initiating event, problem, plans and attempts, consequence, resolution, moral* of story). Progress will be measure using a holistic narrative rating system (see attached). A holistic narrative score will be given to each retelling, with a score of ___ indicating an acceptable narrative (we suggest a target score of approximately 17 of 20 on obligatory features of the narrative rating scale, depending on the child's baseline performance). Criteria for achieving the objective are that the child attains an **acceptable score** on 4 of 6 consecutive retellings (in general, one story per thematic unit is covered approximately every 2 to 3 weeks and a narrative retelling is elicited at the end of each story or thematic unit).

2. Student will demonstrate improved **comprehension** as exhibited by the ability to answer **factual, interpretation** and **inference questions** about stories and expository texts with 80% to 85% accuracy. **Factual** questions are those for which answers are explicitly stated in the text; **interpretation** questions are those for which answers are implied in the text; and **inference** questions are those for which answers are neither implied nor hinted at in the text (reader must utilize background knowledge and reasoning skills to formulate a plausible answer). A set of questions of each type will be generated for each story or expository text, and a rating scale will be used to rate the child's responses. (*Rating scale*: **0** = answer to question was incorrect, implausible; **1** = answer was partially correct, incomplete, possible but not most plausible; **2** = answer was correct, complete, most plausible). A percentage score will be calculated by dividing the total points obtained on the responses to the questions by the total points possible and multiplying by 100.

3. Student will identify, describe, and utilize target **vocabulary** and **concepts** encountered in stories and expository texts (target is the acquisition of **10 to 15 new vocabulary items or concepts per story or thematic unit**). The following rating scale will be used to document the acquisition of new vocabulary and concepts: **0** = child has no concept of the word's meaning, cannot identify or define the word or use it expressively in context; **1** = child has limited or minimal understanding of the word's meaning; may be able to identify it in multiple-choice format or give limited definition, but cannot use the word expressively or spontaneously in context; **2** = child has fully developed understanding of the word's meaning (can identify it receptively, give partial or full definition, may be able to use it in a sentence-formulation task on command) but still does not use the word spontaneously in context; **3** = child has a fully developed concept of the word's meaning, can identify, describe, and define it, as well as use it expressively and spontaneously in context (such as in a narrative-retelling context).

4. Student will identify, explain the formal grammar rule for, and utilize various **grammatical structures, word formation** and **sentence formation** rules (as part of language arts curriculum). Emphasis will be placed on the acquisition and correct use of (choose depending on individual child's needs): **pronouns, noun–verb agreement, regular and irregular plurals, regular and irregular past tense, copula, auxiliary verbs, possessives, compound and complex sentences, use of embedded clauses, negation, interrogatives, punctuation** such as question marks, quotations, semicolons, colons. Progress will be measured by structural analysis of narrative retellings, conversational-speech samples, and written expositions using the following **grammar and morphosyntax scoring system:** **0** = student has no idea what the morphosyntactic element means or how it is used (i.e., cannot explain what the structural element means or how it functions, may not use it correctly in either spoken or written mode); **1** = student has some idea of what the morphosyntactic element means and how it is used (perhaps can explain in limited fashion the formal grammar rule, may be able to perform limited receptive tasks such as fill-in-the-blank or multiple-choice worksheet types of activities involving that morphosyntactic rule or structure), still may not use the structure or rule correctly (expressively) in either spoken or written mode; **2** = student has a more fully developed sense of what the morphosyntactic structure means and how it is used (getting better at explaining the formal grammar rule); the structure may be used correctly (but perhaps still inconsistently) in verbal or written mode; **3** = student has a fully developed sense of what the morphosyntactic structure means and how it is used (can explain the formal grammar rule); the structure is used correctly and consistently in both verbal and written mode.

Box 4-8 Sample Individualized Education Plan Objectives for Literature-Based Intervention—cont'd

5. Student will **read more fluently** and display **multiple strategies for decoding text** (e.g., use of graphophonemic cues, i.e., sound it out, use context and picture clues, semantic clues). Progress will be measured by oral-miscue analysis, rating scales, teacher reporting, rubrics, and other observational or descriptive techniques.

6. Student will use **invented-spelling techniques** and other phonics- and meaning-based strategies to spell new or unfamiliar words during structured writing activities. Progress will be measured by clinician probes, portfolio assessment, rubrics, rating scales, and other observational techniques during completion of actual writing tasks and assignments.

7. Student will **write summary sentences** and **summary paragraphs** about materials read, using the *plan, write, proof, revise* (PWPR) metacognitive strategy. Progress will be measured by clinician probes, portfolio assessment, rubrics, rating scales, and other observational techniques during the completion of actual writing tasks and assignments.

8. Student will engage in the following appropriate **pragmatic** (social communication) behaviors during structured activities, formal classroom discourse, and conversations with peers and teachers.
   - Maintain eye contact; use appropriate body language for situation or context.
   - Engage in message-repair strategies (e.g., repeat, rephrase, paraphrase, provide more information) as needed and on request.
   - Provide sufficient information to the listener.
   - Ask relevant questions and request clarification as needed.
   - Enter into conversations willingly and spontaneously.
   - Initiate, maintain, and switch topics appropriately.
   - Relinquish conversational turn when appropriate; invite others into the conversation.
   - Use appropriate loudness and tone of voice for the context or situation.
   - Express approval or approbation of other students as appropriate during classroom and social situations.
   - Request permission (e.g., for classroom privileges, to borrow or use materials) as appropriate in classroom situations.
   - Observe classroom rules for gaining teacher's attention and answering questions in class (e.g., raise your hand, wait to be recognized before speaking, don't interrupt).
   Progress on these pragmatic objectives are to be measured formally and descriptively by, for example, clinician probes, direct observation, teacher reporting, use of rating scales, and rubrics.

---

the grammar and morphosyntax scoring system (along with other such forms and protocols provided throughout this text) will put some of the critics' concerns to rest.

I also provided a section on the organizational structure and development of expository (informational) text, along with a rationale for the importance of incorporating expository texts into thematic units to support and enhance the language arts curriculum. Finally, I provided a set of detailed IEP goals and objectives for practical use by SLPs and related service providers.

Box 4-9 contains a summary of basic protocol and procedures suggested for literature-based intervention as outlined in this and previous chapters. These procedures may be used consistently or with modifications, with individual clients or with groups, and with multiple stories and thematic units over time.

Box 4-9 Protocol for Literature-Based Intervention

1. Obtain estimates of child's independent, instructional, and frustrational reading grade levels by administering graded reading inventory or other reading battery.
2. Select story for obtaining baseline data. Story should be at child's instructional reading grade level. Use Fry's Readability Graph or other instrument to estimate reading grade level of story.
3. Obtain baseline data:
   a. Have client read story aloud without scaffolding or assistance.
   b. Transcribe and analyze oral-reading miscues (it is best to videotape or audiotape child during oral reading to perform later analysis).
   c. Have client answer series of factual, interpretation, and inference questions about story. Transcribe and score responses later.
   d. Have client retell story in his or her own words (narrative retelling); score narrative retelling using holistic narrative scoring criteria.
4. After analyzing baseline data, begin therapy by rereading same story used during baselining, this time *with* scaffolding. Include thematic art, drama, play, snack, writing, expository text materials, and any supplemental activities as part of thematic unit to support topics and concepts from story.
5. After completing story with scaffolding, repeat data-collection procedures (same as during baseline: oral-reading miscue analysis, response to questions, narrative retelling) for comparison with baseline performance.
6. Begin new story, but this time, scaffold from very beginning (do not have child read story first without scaffolding, as you did with baseline story). When finished with this story, repeat data collection as outlined in step 3. Compare with previous performance.
7. Repeat data-collection procedures at end of each story or thematic unit, or perhaps less often, depending on your schedule (some clinicians prefer to collect data every 6 to 9 weeks for progress notes). With treatment, over time, the following should occur:
   a. Total number of oral-reading miscues should decrease (and qualitative changes in type of miscues may occur, reflecting that child is becoming more balanced strategic reader).
   b. Accuracy on response to factual, interpretation, and inference questions about stories should increase.
   c. Narrative retelling score should improve, and qualitative changes in narrative should occur as well (e.g., improvements in temporality, causality, cohesion, adherence to story grammar elements).

Chapter 5
Building a Power Lexicon: Improving Vocabulary Acquisition in Language-Learning–Disabled Children

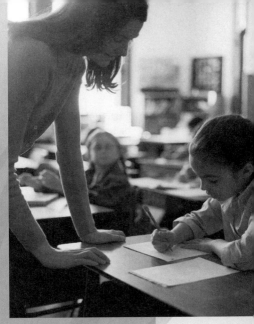

Purposes

- Define what is encompassed by the term *semantics.*
- Review normal lexical and semantic development.
- Describe lexical and semantic difficulties in language-learning–disabled children.
- Discuss the role of vocabulary in reading comprehension and the language arts curriculum.
- Discuss traditional instructional methods for teaching vocabulary versus holistic methods that take advantage of natural acquisition patterns present during early development.

Semantics: More Than Just Vocabulary

According to Baddeley, Gathercole, and Papagno (1998), "learning the vocabulary of one's native language is one of the most important aspects of language acquisition." Furthermore, early childhood represents the most intensive period of new-word learning that humans undergo (Baddeley et al., 1998). Experts have also suggested that vocabulary development may be the "single most important determinant of a child's ultimate academic and intellectual achievements" (Baddeley et al., 1998; Sternberg, 1987). Speech-language pathologists (SLPs) have a long history of paying close attention to vocabulary; indeed, vocabulary is one of the most frequently addressed skills in language therapy and is listed as a goal or objective on practically every language-impaired child's individualized education plan (IEP). However, there is so much more to this domain of language than is typically addressed in traditional language intervention and instructional programs.

Semantics is defined as the "study of meanings in a language, including the analysis of meanings of words, phrases, sentences, discourse, and whole texts" (Harris & Hodges, 1995). As can be seen in this definition, semantics encompasses many meaning-related aspects of language, including what we traditionally think of as vocabulary (i.e., the study of novel words and their definitions). Semantics also incorporates elements such as the following:

- Concept formation (e.g., your concept of what a *dog* is, based on factors such as your perception, experiences, world knowledge)
- Content words of the language (e.g., nouns, verbs, adjectives, adverbs)
- Antonyms, or opposites (e.g., hot/cold; big/little; frightened/brave)
- Synonyms (e.g., cold/cool/chilly; donate/give)
- Multiple meanings such as homonyms, homophones, homographs

There is a great deal of confusion about **homonyms** and how they are defined in the elementary school curriculum and in the linguistics literature. Homonyms are technically defined as "different word meanings converging on the same phonological representation," or "different words having the same name" (Klein & Murphy, 2001). For example, the word *fence* may mean (1) a barrier (sometimes made of wood or wire) intended to prevent escape or intrusion or to mark a boundary; (2) a receiver of stolen goods; (3) a place where stolen goods are bought; (4) to attack or defend with a foil or saber; (5) *on the fence,* a figure of speech used to refer to a position of neutrality or indecision (definitions from *Webster's New Ninth Collegiate Dictionary,* 1990). Likewise, the word *bank* can refer to either a financial institution or the side of a river (Klein & Murphy, 2001).

Polysemy, on the other hand, is defined as "the phenomenon of related senses in otherwise unambiguous words, such as object/substance, object/representation of that object, type/token, and text/object containing that text. . . . certain semantic relations between a word's senses may appear over and over in polysemy" (Klein & Murphy, 2001).

An example of a polysemous word would be *paper,* which may be used to refer to "a substance made of wood pulp, a blank sheet of that substance, a daily news publication, an article printed on that substance," or perhaps even "a student's 'paper' turned in electronically or on computer disk such that wood pulp is in no way involved" (Klein & Murphy, 2001). In this example, the different senses of the word *paper*, though all

semantically related to some extent, are dependent on the context of use.

Linguists continue to disagree about how homonymous and polysemous words are represented in the lexicon (i.e., in the brain); this theoretical matter has important implications later as we explore treatment for lexical difficulties in the language-learning–disabled (LLD) population. For the practicing SLP, the issue of homonymous and polysemous words can best be summarized as having to do with *situations in which a word can have more than one meaning, based on context.* We can also be sure that we will encounter many instances in which LLD children are confused about the meaning of a homonymous or polysemous word because they cannot distinguish its meaning based on context.

Other elements of semantics include:

- Categorization (superordinate and subordinate categories, e.g., *furniture = chair, sofa, table, desk, bed*); learning the **prototype** or best examplar of a word or category and then learning less typical examplars (e.g., *chair = high chair, rocking chair, kitchen table chair, child's chair, easy chair, desk chair, leather chair, upholstered chair*)
- **Semantic features**—that is, aspects of meaning that characterize a word (e.g., *dog = has four legs, barks, wears a collar, wags its tail, walks on a leash*)
- **Selective restrictions** that prohibit certain word combinations because they are meaningless or redundant (e.g., *male mother, hot snow*)
- Vocabulary (definitions, both denotative and connotative meanings)
- Whole-sentence meanings

Sentences represent a meaning greater than the sum of the individual words that make up that sentence; listeners and readers tend to focus on whole-sentence meaning, and to do that, they must readily understand relationships between and across the words in the sentence.

As can be seen from the previous summary, semantics includes what we traditionally think of as vocabulary but also encompasses broader aspects of meaning in the language. Unfortunately, too many SLPs and regular and special educators have failed to recognize this fact and have also failed to take into account the myriad and often subtle deficits that LLD children display across and throughout the semantic domain.

Lexical Acquisition

The **lexicon** may be defined as "a person's mental dictionary" or the "sum of the words he or she knows and uses." The question of how we develop our lexicon and learn new words and their meanings has fascinated psycholinguists and other experts for many years and continues to stir lively debate.

From birth until entering school, children learn new words and word meanings primarily through context and immersion—that is, through exposure to verbal interactions in their environment (Kamhi & Catts, 1991; Throneburg, Calvert, Sturm, Paramboukas, & Paul, 2000). That is why exposure to a rich language environment during a child's formative years is so important. On entering school, children still learn new words through context and immersion, but emphasis is now also placed on teaching children new vocabulary formally, through various modes of instruction. During elementary school, and by third grade in particular, reading becomes the primary method of vocabulary exposure and acquisition (Nagy & Anderson, 1984). The best methods for teaching vocabulary formally, however, remain a subject of lively and spirited debate in educational circles. Throneburg et al.

(2000) note that "future investigation of the SLP's role in facilitating vocabulary learning, reading comprehension, and curricular success is necessary after third grade." As noted previously, third grade poses a critical milestone for students; it is when the curriculum makes the transition from *learning to read* to *reading to learn*. Exploring the SLP's role in facilitating vocabulary acquisition, particularly through reading, is one of the primary goals of this chapter.

First, however, I will describe the sequence of normal lexical development in young children (Box 5-1). The toddler and preschool period is characterized by rapid lexical growth (sometimes referred to as the *vocabulary growth spurt*). It is estimated that a child adds approximately 9 or 10 words to his or her lexicon daily (Carey, 1978), although in reality, this impressive statistic really refers to the child's rate of **fast-mapping**, or "the representation of a new word on the basis of a few incidental exposures" (McGregor, Friedman, Reilly, & Newman, 2002). Studies also show that reading to children frequently from a young age has a tremendously positive impact on their developing lexicons.

It has been suggested that word learning may actually be a two-part process. Part 1 is fast-mapping, whereby the child infers a connection between a word and its referent in as little as one exposure (Pinker, 1982). This fast-mapping is probably largely receptive at first, and the actual amount of information the child stores about the word on

---

Box 5-1 Review of Normal Semantic and Lexical Development

12 months	First true words
18 months	Begins to use 2-word utterances; has approx. 20-word vocabulary
24 months	Has 200- to 300-word vocabulary; names most common everyday objects
3 years	Has 900- to 1,000-word vocabulary
4 years	Has 1500- to 1600-word vocabulary; categorizes; relies on word order for interpretation (semantics and syntax intricately related)
5 years	Has 2100- to 2200-word vocabulary
6 years	Has expressive vocabulary of 2600 words, receptive vocabulary of 20,000 to 24,000 words; defines by function; uses all parts of speech to some degree; beginning to understand abstract and figurative language
8 years	Very verbal; expresses ideas and problems readily
12 years	Has 50,000-word expressive vocabulary; constructs adultlike definitions
18 years	Has meanings for 80,000 words

Modified from Language Development: An Introduction *by R. Owens, 1996, (4th ed.), Boston: Allyn & Bacon; and from "How children learn words," by G. A. Miller, & P. M. Gildea, 1987, Scientific American, 257, 94–99.*

initial exposure is variable (based on previous word and world knowledge). Part 2 of word learning is thought to be characterized by an extended phase in which the child gradually refines the rough definition of the word, based on subsequent encounters (i.e., with repeated exposure, the child acquires more semantic features of the word and gradually refines the definition). Carey (1978) referred to this extended word-learning phase as *slow-mapping,* a period when the child must "hold a fragile new representation in lexical memory, distinguish it from many other fragile representations, continue to hypothesize about the meaning of the word, and update representations as a result of those hypotheses (McGregor et al., 2002). McGregor et al. note that in reality, the extended phase of word learning might take "weeks, months, or years, depending on the semantic complexity and frequency of the word to be learned." So rather than 10 new words a day, what children may really be learning is "one-hundredth of each of a thousand different words" (Bloom, 2000). Clearly, there is much more to this word-learning business than we thought! As the child's lexicon expands, there is a need for increased organization, and semantic networks and interrelationships between words and concepts are formed (Owens, 1996).

Based on the idea of fast-mapping (i.e., that word learning does not take place all at once, and that there may be levels or gradations of word knowledge as a new lexical entry is integrated into the child's semantic network through repeated exposures over time), the continuum shown in Box 5-2 may be useful when one is attempting to conceptualize an individual's level of mastery of a particular lexical item.

Late Talkers and Slow Expressive Language Development

It is important to note that the generally accepted definition of a *late talker* is a child who has an expressive vocabulary of less than 50 words at 24 months of age, and/or one who is not beginning to put two words together into short utterances by the same age (Rescorla, 1989). It is estimated that approximately 10% to 15% of middle-class American children may fit this late-talker profile and that somewhere between 75% to 80% of them will outgrow the problem spontaneously (Owens,

---

Box 5-2 Word Knowledge Continuum

0 = Individual has no knowledge of meaning of word and cannot or does not use it expressively

1 = Individual has limited knowledge of meaning of word (may have picked up some cues from hearing or reading word in context and may exhibit this knowledge in receptive modality, such as pointing to picture to match word or choosing correct definition in multiple-choice format); cannot or does not use word expressively.

2 = Individual has fairly well developed knowledge of meaning of word (e.g., may be able to give partial definition on command); beginning to use word expressively (e.g., may be able to use word in simple sentence on command).

3 = Individual has fully developed knowledge of meaning of word (gives full definition); uses word spontaneously and appropriately in expressive mode.

1999). For the approximately 20% to 25% of these late talkers who do not catch up to their peers in the area of expressive language (i.e., those exhibiting *slow expressive language development,* or *expressive language delay*), the problem is expected to persist through preschool into the school-age years, developing into a more specific language problem (Paul, 1989, 1996; Rescorla, 1990). Note that estimates of the percentage of late talkers who spontaneously recover vary, and research in this area is continuing. Research suggests that children with expressive language delay appear to have persisting problems in the areas of syntax and phonology, even after they have apparently caught up to their normal-language peers in other areas (Paul, 1993).

It is also interesting to note that lexical acquisition is one of the few areas of language that is not *quite* as constrained by the confines of the critical period. We can and do continue to learn new words throughout our lives, albeit not as rapidly as we did during the critical period of language acquisition, when our brains were maximally flexible and primed for learning new words. The amount of lexical acquisition that occurs in the adolescent and adult years depends a great deal on contextual variables such as our educational levels, the occupations we choose, our lifestyles, how avid readers we are, and whether or not we make a conscious effort to continue learning new words on a daily basis.

Definitions—An Area of Avid Devotion in the Language Arts Curriculum

How many of you remember getting a list of vocabulary words from your elementary school teacher at the beginning of the week, being required to look up and write down the definitions of those words, and then spending hours memorizing definitions so that you could be tested on those words or definitions at the end of the week? For many children this still constitutes the way formal vocabulary is taught in the language arts curriculum: a list of isolated words separated from any meaningful context is presented to the students, who are then expected to memorize the words and definitions, and somehow add those items to their productive lexicons. Besides being boring and repetitive, this instructional paradigm seldom achieves the desired result. Rarely do the children transfer these lexical items and definitions to their productive lexicons—you seldom if ever hear them using the new words in their spontaneous discourse nor do you see them using the words in their written narratives or paragraph summaries. So why do we keep doing it this way? I have never been given a satisfactory answer to that question by administrators and curriculum planners, even when I point out that all research and practical evidence suggests that this is the least facilitative instructional method for teaching vocabulary.

It is interesting to me that despite such avid devotion to vocabulary and definitions in the elementary school language arts curriculum, very few educators, administrators, or SLPs seem to be familiar with the normal development sequence of definitional abilities in children.

Definitional Abilities in Children

It is generally assumed that as a child's word knowledge accumulates he or she may choose the correct definition of a word from several alternatives but still may not be able to express the meaning of the word spontaneously (Johnson & Anglin,

1995). Eventually, as knowledge of a particular word grows (i.e., during the extended phase of word learning), the child will be able to express the word's meaning in the form of a verbal definition. According to Johnson and Anglin (1995), it is this ability to produce an explicit high-quality verbal definition that is generally accepted as evidence that a particular lexical item has been mastered and is now available for language use. It is for this reason that so many IQ tests and standardized language instruments require subjects to provide verbal definitions (Johnson & Anglin, 1995). Likewise, being able to provide high-quality definitions is considered to be a strong correlate of literacy attainment and academic success (Chall, 1987; Johnson & Anglin, 1995).

In a landmark study published in 1993, Anglin investigated school-age children's definitional abilities by examining their knowledge of a large sample of words shown to be representative of the contents of an unabridged dictionary (representative in terms of both word frequency and the relative distribution of various morphological types). Anglin credited both the children's receptive understanding of the words (i.e., multiple-choice format corrected for guessing) and expressed word knowledge (i.e., definitional attempts). Anglin then estimated total word knowledge by multiplying the proportion of sample words known by the 258,601 total words in the dictionary. Results yielded estimates of "dramatic vocabulary growth" during the elementary school years: from 10,398 known words in first grade to 39,994 words in fifth grade (Anglin, 1993).

Johnson and Anglin further analyzed children's definitional attempts (specifically, expressed word knowledge) in a study published in 1995. This study allowed the authors to (1) estimate the number of words for which children of different ages could provide definitions of varied quality and (2) compare the quality of definitions provided for various parts of speech (e.g., noun, verb, adjective) and for various morphological compositions (e.g., root, compound, inflected, derived). Johnson and Anglin began their article with an excellent review of the literature summarizing information regarding definitional abilities and studies to date. Box 5-3 summarizes some of the important information from their very thorough literature review. Readers are urged to refer to the Johnson and

---

Box 5-3 What We Know About Definitions: A Review of the Literature

- A *high-quality definition* generally serves as both a semantic and a syntactic *substitute* for the word being defined.
- A definition expresses the meaning of the word in a *synonymous*, alternative form that can *take the place of* the target word in a sentence.
- Being able to provide a definition requires engaging in *metalinguistic operations*.
- A definition generally incorporates precise semantic content and is phrased in terms general enough to include most uses of the word yet *specific enough to distinguish that word's meaning from those of semantically related concepts*.
- A definition adheres to conventional syntactical form when it matches the part of speech of the target word being defined (e.g., verb-phrase definition for a target verb being defined; noun-phrase definition for a target noun being defined).
- Verb and adjective definitions tend to be more variable in form than noun definitions, and the development of verb and adjective definitions has not been studied as extensively as noun definitions.
- Development of definitional abilities proceeds gradually along form and content dimensions; however, change in one dimension is not necessarily linked to changes in the other. Children eventually learn to coordinate both form and content within the definition.
- Many words that are known receptively cannot be defined easily, even by adults (because of the nature and complexity of the words themselves). For instance, concrete nouns (e.g., house, car) are easier to define than abstract nouns (e.g., pleasure, art). Definitional skills for verbs and adjectives develop later than those for nouns, perhaps because they are less easy to define.
- The mental lexicon appears to be organized differently for nouns, verbs, and adjectives, and this may also affect definitional abilities.
- What goes on during the fast-mapping and extended word-learning phases is still not completely understood; as children go through the gradual and protracted process of elaborating and reorganizing word knowledge, their definitional skills are also affected in ways we still don't completely understand.
- Many studies of children's definitions have focused on nouns in root-word form. However, the majority of lexical entries in unabridged dictionaries consist of morphologically complex forms (i.e., derived words, inflected words, and literal compounds). More research is needed in this area.

Modified from "Qualitative Developments in the Content and Form of Children's Definitions," *by C. J. Johnson and J. M. Anglin, 1995,* Journal of Speech-Language-Hearing Research, 38, 612-629.

Anglin article for a complete summation of their literature review and research findings.

As previously indicated, Johnson and Anglin decided to extend the results of Anglin's 1993 study by exploring the expressed word knowledge of 96 children (32 each in first, third, and fifth grades) from two elementary schools in Ontario. Words were selected from a large unabridged dictionary by sampling every seventh entry from every sixth page. The sampling list was judged to be representative in terms of word frequency and morphological word types found in the dictionary. Word knowledge was assessed by having the children participate in as many as three tasks (administered in a hierarchy of decreasing difficulty) including (1) defining the word verbally, (2) using the word in a sentence to show knowledge of its meaning, or (3) recognizing the word's meaning from among four alternatives. The children's definitions were then classified according to both the quality of the semantic content and the syntactical form.

Results revealed that the school-age children showed "considerable growth in expressed word knowledge" as revealed by the quality of their definitional responses to the sample words from the unabridged dictionary. With development the children not only gave definitions for greater numbers of words, but their definitions met higher-quality standards for both form and content (i.e., semantics and morphosyntax), lending credence to the theory that definitional skill represents the "eventual coordination of separately developing semantic and syntactic knowledge" (Johnson & Anglin, 1995).

Johnson and Anglin's study also provided a much better picture of the actual changes in word knowledge that occurred between grades one and five. Their vocabulary growth estimates varied greatly depending on the level of word knowledge assessed—that is, the quality of the children's definitions and the criteria that were used to judge the definitions (see the article for a detailed description of the rating scale used to judge the quality of the children's definitions). For definitions judged as *high quality*, estimates of the children's word knowledge increased from 259 words in first grade to 5689 words in fifth grade. For all levels of word knowledge (i.e., not necessarily high-quality definitions but also lower-quality definitions), estimates ranged from 6145 in first grade to 25,361 words in fifth grade. For expressed knowledge combined with receptive knowledge (assessed by the multiple-choice format), estimates ranged from 10,398 in first grade to 39,994 words in fifth grade.

In summary, what this study confirmed is that children undergo substantial growth in vocabulary during the elementary school years, but that the growth estimates vary considerably according to the criteria of what we purport to be measuring (e.g., receptive and expressed word knowledge versus expressed word knowledge only). Most importantly, how we judge expressed word knowledge and the criteria or level of stringency we set for what constitutes a high-quality definition makes a tremendous difference in our estimates of vocabulary growth across grade levels. This has serious ramifications for the SLP, who lists vocabulary as part of the goals and objectives on practically every IEP. Seldom do I see these issues addressed in the IEP objective for vocabulary and lexical acquisition. We must ask, What are we striving for with these children? Receptive word knowledge? Expressed word knowledge? Both? If so, how will this knowledge be attained and measured? Through verbal definitions? Through multiple-choice format? Some sort of task hierarchy similar to the one used in the Johnson and Anglin study? (A good idea, by the way! The Johnson and Anglin system for measuring expressed word knowledge is valid, reliable, and easy to use, and it is the practicing SLP's failure to specify how mastery of the vocabulary goals and objectives will be measured that is a big part of the problem. If a system designed by researchers works, why not apply it during real therapy?). What about the developmental continuum along the way

(i.e., some of the milestones that children must achieve before they can produce a high-quality definition that coordinates both content and form)? Are we taking all that into consideration in our treatment planning and intervention? I find that many SLPs are simply unaware of these important semantic considerations. We simply must become better informed and be clear about what it is we are expecting children to do in the domain of semantics and vocabulary. We cannot afford to neglect vocabulary, definitions, and semantics; we simply must be better educated about these linguistic domains ourselves before we can engage in effective curricular planning and intervention.

Box 5-4 contains a brief review of the sequence of development of definitional abilities in children (this one is designed to share with parents and teachers, because it contains the bare essentials).

What About Lexicon Acquisition in Language-Learning–Disabled Children?

Difficulties

LLD children often exhibit a variety of difficulties in the area of semantics and vocabulary development (Box 5-5), but difficulty adding new words to their lexicon is an important one and obviously an area deserving our attention. If I had to sum up LLD children's semantic deficits (based on my years of working with them as a school-based SLP working in pull-out and classroom-based contexts), I would have to say that they exhibit limited variety and flexibility of word usage and an impoverished lexicon. Obviously they have difficulty learning new words in the traditional ways they are taught and presented in school (i.e., being given isolated lists of vocabulary words and being expected to look up the definitions and memorize them). With their limited spelling abilities, looking up words in a dictionary is problematic for school-age LLD children (they often do not understand how to use the dictionary and lack alphabetization skills, which are highly phonologically dependent in the first place). Their reading deficits make it highly improbable that they will be able to decipher a structured definition they find in the dictionary, and their short- and long-term memory deficits make it that much harder to commit such a

---

Box 5-4 Sequence of Development for Definitional Abilities in Children

Toddler and Preschool Years

Child first learns prototype and most common examplar of a word or category, based on perceptual knowledge and experiences with the world (e.g., *chair* refers to all chairs—easy chair, rocking chair, high chair, desk chair, etc.). Child is generally unable to give a formal dictionary-type definition: he or she is much more likely to identify perceptual attributes or semantic features of the word, object, or category or state or demonstrate the function. However, some children as young as 3 years of age can provide a verbal definition of sorts that includes function, physical, and locative properties of objects; it may occasionally include categorical information.

School-Age Years

Definition acquires more semantic features of the prototype; definitions become less based on individual perception and experience and more based on socially shared meaning. Child is usually able to give a simple definition of a word or object or category if it is in his or her lexicon; definition often consists of listing semantic features, a description of function, maybe synonyms.

Adolescence

Definitions improve quantitatively and qualitatively; synonym-type definitions increase; there is a greater tendency to include categorical membership, function, description, and degree in the definition.

Adult

Definitions tend to be abstract and descriptive and include concrete terms or references or give specific examples or instances; the definitions use synonyms, explanations, and categorizations of the word defined; they may also be exclusionary, that is, specify what an entity is *not*.

Modified from "Cups and Glasses: Learning That Boundaries Are Vague," by E. S. Anderson, 1975, Journal of Child Language, 2, 79–103; *"Qualitative Developments in the Content and Form of Children's Definitions" by C. J. Johnson, and J. M. Anglin, 1995,* Journal of Speech-Language-Hearing Research, 38, 612–629; *"Semantic Representation in Young Children," by K. K. McGregor, R. M. Friedman, R. M. Reilly, and R. M. Newman, 2002,* Journal of Speech, Language and Hearing Research, 45, 332–346; *and* Language Development: An Introduction *(4th ed.), by R. Owens, 1996, Boston: Allyn & Bacon.*

definition to memory. Finally, even if they are able to commit a definition to memory, there is certainly no guarantee that they will transfer the novel word and its meaning to their receptive and productive lexicon (i.e., they may be unsuccessful in enmeshing the new word into their intricate and delicate network of previous word and world knowledge). As we have seen, true mastery of a word and all its shades of meaning is a gradual process that requires repeated exposure to the target word in multiple, meaningful contexts, and if this is true for normal-language learners, it is perhaps more so for LLD learners.

Implications

Because vocabulary is a major component of the elementary school language arts curriculum, semantic and lexical deficits can have a dramatic negative impact on communication and academic performance in school-age children. Research also suggests that vocabulary instruction may have a significant effect on children's comprehension of text (so vocabulary and reading comprehension are inextricably linked). However, there is still controversy about the best way to teach vocabulary to school-age children and how to remediate vocabulary deficits in LLD children.

Research suggests that the most effective vocabulary teaching methods are the following:

1. Include both a definitional and a contextual component.
2. Involve the students in deeper processing of the new words.
3. Give students more than one exposure to the to-be-learned words (Stahl & Fairbanks, 1986).

Literature-based intervention, using scaffolded interaction (e.g., *communicative reading strategies* Norris, 1988, 1989, 1991, 1992) meets all these criteria.

Box 5-5 Lexical and Semantic Deficits in Language-Learning–Disabled Children

- Delayed receptive and expressive vocabulary (often late talkers; do not add words with rapidity during ages 1 to 3 years, when most children are adding new words rapidly)
- Difficulty learning new vocabulary and definitions of words (and failure to generalize use of such words and definitions into their expressive language)
- Limited variety and flexibility of word use or limited lexical diversity (as measured by type/token ratio)
- Difficulty with abstract and figurative vocabulary and nonliteral meanings (e.g., idioms, metaphors, similes.)
- Anomia or word-retrieval difficulties (with accompanying circumlocutions and interjections or fillers)
- Particular difficulty with verbs (now considered a hallmark of Specific Language Impairment)
- Difficulty inferring word meanings from contextual cues
- Lack of strategies for looking up words in the dictionary; can not decipher definition if they do manage to look it up

What Is the Goal of Lexicon and Vocabulary Acquisition?

The goal of vocabulary acquisition for proficient language users should be to build a rich, varied, and powerful lexicon. And by *rich*, we don't just mean *big* (although it certainly doesn't hurt to know plenty of words!). It is not just a matter of how many words we know, but how elaborated our semantic network is (i.e., how many semantic features we have for a word and how well connected words are to each other by association in our lexicon). A person with a rich, powerful lexicon exhibits variety and flexibility of word use— that person's language will likely be dynamic, vibrant, and interesting because of lexical diversity.

According to J. Norris (personal communication, September 1994), the focus of language intervention should be on teaching *process*, not *product*. By focusing on processes and strategies, the clinician will not only help the child learn something truly useful, but "will also end up getting good 'product'

into the bargain anyway" (J. Norris, personal communication, September 1994). Applied to the area of semantic intervention, our goal should be not to just add words to the child's lexicon (like adding pennies to a piggy bank); rather, our goal should be to teach the child multiple strategies for processing new vocabulary that he or she encounters in context (e.g., in written texts, spoken dialogue, classroom discourse). If the child (1) masters the strategies for deciphering new word meanings from context, (2) learns to use reference tools such as dictionaries and thesauri to locate additional information on word meanings, and (3) obtains repeated exposure and practice with the novel word or words in multiple contexts over time, then the product of intervention will be the addition of new vocabulary anyway. More importantly, the child will not just master the vocabulary encountered in a single lesson from a language arts textbook, or a single list of words or definitions that is presented at the beginning of the week in class and then tested for mastery on Friday. The child who has truly mastered meaning-based strategies will be successful at adding new words and concepts throughout life. In this case, mastery of *process = product*.

Suggestions for Therapy and Instruction

Box 5-6 contains a list of suggestions that SLPs may wish to incorporate into the semantic and lexical intervention process for building a well-connected powerful lexicon in LLD children.

Vocabulary and Classroom Collaboration

A 2000 study by Throneburg et al. compared the effectiveness of three different service-delivery models for improving the curricular vocabulary of a group of normal and speech-language–impaired children in kindergarten through third grade. The three approaches were (1) a collaborative approach (SLP and teacher team-teach), (2) a classroom-based approach (with the SLP and teacher working separately and independently in the classroom), and (3) a traditional pull-out approach. Results indicated that the collaborative team-teaching model

---

Box 5-6 Suggestions for Semantic and Lexical Intervention

- Teach the *metalinguistic* aspects of vocabulary acquisition (e.g., show how to learn new words and their meanings, discuss and explore the advantages of having a rich and powerful vocabulary in day-to-day life).
- Provide exposure and experience with *various literary genres* (i.e., narratives and fictional storybooks, magazines, various types of expository texts such as textbooks, nonfiction books, encyclopedias, almanacs, drama and plays, poetry). These various genres contain rich, diverse vocabulary already embedded in a meaningful context.
- Teach the child how to make deductions and inferences about word meanings based on *context*.
- But still teach the child how to *look up definitions* in a dictionary and how to decipher the definitional dictionary entry (and don't forget all the wonderful options available on computers such as on-line dictionary, thesaurus, encyclopedia).
- Focus not just on teaching new words and their meanings, but on *enmeshing* or *intertwining* new words into the child's existing lexicon to create a rich, *elaborated semantic network* (note that this works as both *top-down* and *bottom-up* processing by urging the child to use his or her prior word or world knowledge to help figure out meanings of new words, as well as to attach or hook new words to items already existing in the child's lexicon).
- Explore *collaborative-consultation* service delivery models that elicit a teacher's input about curricular vocabulary and semantic goals, which will ensure academic relevance (Throneburg et al., 2000).

---

was most effective for teaching curricular vocabulary to children who qualified for speech-language therapy services, and that SLPs can have a positive impact on vocabulary growth of all students in a classroom (including those who do not qualify for speech-language therapy services) when using a collaborative or classroom-based model. SLPs should be proactive about using alternative service-delivery models for intervening in the arena of semantics, as well as other aspects of the language arts curriculum (see Chapter 7 for further details on implementing alternative service-delivery models and suggestions for classroom collaboration).

Literature As an Authentic Context for Vocabulary Instruction

Rupley, Logan, and Nichols (1999) indicate that vocabulary instruction should take a prominent role in any balanced reading program. They recommend an eclectic approach in which both wide reading and direct instructional techniques are used to promote vocabulary acquisition. As always, instruction should focus on connecting new lexical items to words and concepts the student already knows in order to create a well-connected, flexible lexicon. Rupley et al. recommend providing students with ample opportunities to discuss and elaborate on the meanings of new words, along with multiple opportunities to use the new words outside the text in which they were encountered. Obviously, all these principles of instruction fit nicely with the kind of scaffolded dialogue and literature-based intervention I have discussed throughout this textbook so far. Box 5-7 provides the dialogue from a session that illustrates some of these principles.

It is important to note that some of the key vocabulary items discussed in the dialogue in Box 5-7 were never directly mentioned in the story *Jim's Trumpet*. That again is one of the beauties of literature-based intervention. The text facilitates you, gives you ideas and a starting point for instruction and intervention, but you are by no means bound by the text. Not only is it possible to explore vocabulary directly encountered in the text (see Box 4-3 for specific vocabulary items targeted in *Jim's Trumpet*), but by building a thematic unit, the students and teacher or clinician are often able to pull in even more relevant, thematically related vocabulary (e.g., in this case the terms *urban, suburban,* and associated terminology to describe lifestyles in those settings) (Table 5-1).

Using Dictionary Skills to Build a Rich and Powerful Lexicon With Language-Learning–Disabled Children

As previously mentioned, a balanced vocabulary program should include both a wide reading component (i.e., scaffolded dialogue and extension activities while the student is reading authentic literature in a variety of genres) and a formal definition

Box 5-7   Transcript of Session for Thematic Unit on Urban Versus Suburban Living After Reading *Jim's Trumpet*

Students. Students are in fourth and fifth grade, age 10 to 11—years, three enrolled in self-contained special-education class for learning-disabled students. All three students receive speech-language therapy for receptive and expressive language deficits. All three students read significantly below chronological or grade level expectancies.

Context or activity. Clinician and students have been reading the story *Jim's Trumpet* and building a thematic unit around that story for several sessions.

C: Let's continue our discussion about Jim and where he lived. Let's look at the cover of the book again for clues. Where did Jim live?

P: In an apartment building, in the city?

C: Yes, it appears from the picture that Jim lives in an apartment building, probably in the city. The apartment building appears to have several *stories* or *floors*. How do we know that?

S: Because he was sitting on the fire escape playin his music. That's that stair thing outside the building, so the people can ekscape (dialectal variation) if there's a fire.

C: That's right! So if there are multiple stairs or levels on the fire escape, Jim must live in a *high-rise* building. You usually see those in the city, right?

(All students nod and/or say, "Um hmm" to indicate agreement.)

C: So, we agree that from the evidence in the picture and the text, that Jim lives in the city. There's a new vocabulary word I want to introduce today. It's a word that means "having to do with the city." That word is *urban*. (Clinician writes the word on the dry-erase board.) Any of you heard that word before?

(Students shake their heads to indicate "no.")

C: Well, maybe we had better look it up in the dictionary then, just to clarify the definition. S., could you get the dictionary for us?

(S. gets children's dictionary.)

C: Can you look up *urban* for us?

(S. struggles with looking up the word; it is apparent that she cannot use the tabs on the sides of the pages or alphabetized guide words at the top of the pages.)

C: Do you all remember how to look up words in the dictionary? What do we use at the top of the pages to guide us?

U: Guide words?

C: Yes! U., can you explain to S. how to use guide words?

U: You gotta look for a guide word that starts with the same letters as the word you wanna look up. So look for words at the top that start with *u-r*.

C: That's correct. U., go ahead and help S.

(U. helps S. turn to the correct section of the dictionary using the alphabetized tabs on the sides of the pages and guide words at the top of the page; C. then helps them both scan down the page to locate the entry *urban*.)

C: Here it is! S., could you read the definition for us?

S: of, relating to or char-char-(struggling to decode).

C: charact-(giving a bit more of a phonemic cue).

S: (continues) characteristic of a city.

C: So we were correct. *Urban* means "characteristic of," or "having to do with a city." For instance, a person who lives in a city is sometimes referred to as an *urban dweller* (writing this phrase on the board under *urban*). And when people tear down old buildings and rebuild them, that is sometimes referred to as *urban renewal* (writing down that phrase). But let's focus our thoughts today on what it means to be an urban dweller, because that's what Jim is. He's an urban dweller, someone who lives in the city, right?

(Students all nod affirmatively.)

C: Now, Jim doesn't *remain* an urban dweller for the entire story does he? Seems like I recall from our reading that he moved somewhere else for a brief time. Who remembers where? P., do you remember?

P: He went to live with his sister? In another part of town?

C: That's true. Let's look at that picture (turns to appropriate page in the book). Look at Jim's sister's house and the surrounding yard. Does it look like *she* is an *urban dweller*?

---

*C, Clinician; S, female student; U, male student; P, male student.

Continued

Box 5-7 Transcript of Session for Thematic Unit on Urban Versus Suburban Living After Reading *Jim's Trumpet*—cont'd

No. It look like she live out in the country.

C: Are you sure? Out in the *country*? I don't see any cows, or horses, or fields or crops growing!

P: (Laughs.) Not the country, I mean like out where *we* live. . . . not, not the city, but, in a regular neighborhood.

C: Yes! Not in the big city exactly, but not way out in the country either! There's a name for that kind of place too! It's called a *suburb* (writing word on board). If you live in a *suburb*, it means a smaller city located next to a big city, or a neighborhood just outside the big city.

P: Like Marrero is to New Orleans!

C: That's right! Marrero is a smaller city next to a big city. It is a *suburb*. And you are all *suburban dwellers*.

(Students all laugh, indicating that they get it.)

C: See how the two words look next to each other (writes *urban* and *suburban* next to each other). Look, *urban* is the root word, and *sub* is the prefix! And *sub* means a lesser or smaller part, right? So since *urban* refers to "city," then *suburban* must refer to a "smaller version of a city." Right?

(Students nod.)

C: You know, I wonder how Jim liked that change—moving from the big city to the surburbs? I wonder what was different about it? Besides playing his trumpet in his building, do you suppose there were *other things* he missed about being an *urban dweller*? Things he could only do in the big city, that he couldn't do out in the suburbs at his sister's house?

(Students' facial affect indicates interest in the topic.)

C: Why don't we make a *comparison-contrast chart* (Table 5-1) to show what would be different about living in the big city, versus living in a suburb or regular neighborhood? I'd be interested to hear your opinions—would you rather be an urban dweller or a suburban dweller, and why?

S: Oooh—when I grow up I wanna live in the *Big* city!

C: You do? Why? What is better about being an urban dweller?

(Students and clinician went on to generate a chart similar to the one in Table 5-1.)

*C, Clinician; *S,* female student; *U,* male student; *P,* male student.

Table 5-1 Sample Comparison and Contrast Chart Generated by Language-Learning–Disabled Group and Clinician for Urban Versus Suburban Living (Part of Thematic Unit for *Jim's Trumpet*)

URBAN OR BIG-CITY LIVING	SUBURBAN LIVING
High-rise buildings, skyscrapers, apartments, less space, more crowded	Houses, yards, some apartments, more space, less crowded
Mass transportation (bus, taxi, train, subway), traffic	Cars, some traffic (not as much as city)
Museums, restaurants, nightclubs, theaters	Shopping malls, some restaurants, movie theaters
Schools (smaller playgrounds? But maybe a better band, more school clubs, better field trips, more extracurricular activities and things to do in the city on weekends?)	Schools (bigger playgrounds? But maybe not as good of a band, fewer school clubs, not as many interesting field trips or things to do outside of school on weekends?)
More crime (have to be very careful)	Less crime (but still have to be careful)
More jobs (people often move or have to relocate to a city because of jobs)	Fewer jobs (people often prefer to live in the suburbs but still have to commute to the city for their jobs)

and dictionary component. Accordingly, the following are some suggestions for working with the dictionary and teaching dictionary skills to LLD students:

- Whenever possible, use words from the grade-level curriculum or thematic units or directly from texts (fiction or expository) to look up in a dictionary, rather than random words that were not originally embedded in a meaningful context.
- Keep a children's dictionary and thesaurus handy during all therapy sessions (one for each child in the group if possible).
- Explain the alphabetical system, use of indented tabs or other alphabetized dividers (generally on the sides of the pages), and use of guide words (at the top of each page in the dictionary) for looking up words in the dictionary. Provide lots of practice using the alphabetized system, and design games with prizes for looking up words for a particular thematic unit (e.g., if you are doing a thematic unit on sea life, create game boards and use the dictionary to locate words as you move along the board—perhaps, "Who can find me a word that starts with the letters *m-o-r* that means "a type of eel?").
- Explain the parts of a dictionary entry (e.g., the pronunciation key, the etymology or origin of the word [if given], how the prototypical definition is often given first, with less likely definitions following in sequence).
- Explain any other abbreviations relating to usage and parts of speech (e.g., functional labels such as *n.* means noun, *v.* means verb).
- Show how a word is used in a sentence in the dictionary entry to help illustrate its meaning (it is a good idea to have the child make up another sentence with the same word to see if the child really got the definition).
- Don't forget to put any words you extracted from the text and looked up in the dictionary back into their original context. Otherwise looking up words is just an exercise in futility and children rarely see the point of it. Do this by having the student reread the part of the text where the word you looked up originally came from and discuss the nuances of meaning that

you gleaned from looking up the word in the dictionary in relation to how the word is used in its authentic literary context (e.g., paraphrase, summarize).

- To explore the concept of synonyms and use of a thesaurus, take a sample paragraph from a storybook or expository text and highlight key words for which you want the child to find a synonym in the thesaurus (make a photocopy if you do not wish to alter the original book). Then have the child locate the highlighted words in the thesaurus. Cross out the highlighted words in the original text, have the child write the synonyms above the original words, and then reread the paragraph using the synonyms. (This task is also easily done on the computer using Microsoft Word—the clinician and child can simply word-process a short piece of the text on the computer and use the colored highlight or colored font and strikethrough functions to make the necessary changes. Children often find it fun to use the computer in this fashion as well, so it adds an incentive for engaging in the task). Be sure to discuss how using the synonyms slightly changes the meaning of the paragraph compared with the meaning when the original words were used.
- Show how using synonyms can eliminate redundancy (i.e., use of the same word over and over in adjacent sentences or in a paragraph).
- Use paraphrasing and synonyms when discussing literature to solidify the meaning of new vocabulary and concepts and to build lexical diversity (e.g., "Yes, the giant was *very angry* when Jack ran away with the goose that laid golden eggs and the magical harp. I would be *furious* too if someone stole such valuable things from me.").

Individualized Education Plan Goals And Objectives

As before, I conclude with a list of suggested IEP goals and objectives that are in keeping with the suggestions made in this chapter (Box 5-8). These can easily be modified to suit the individual needs of the student and/or clinician.

Summary

In this chapter we have discovered that children learn new words primarily through context and immersion in the language of their environment during their toddler and preschool years. Word learning appears to be a two-part process (the ini-tial phase is called *fast-mapping* and is followed by an extended, gradual phase of learning whereby more features and nuances of meaning are added and the word is intertwined into the individual's complex network of previous world and word knowledge). This latter stage may take days, months, or years, depending on the characteristics

---

Box 5-8 Goals and Objectives for Semantics and Lexical Acquisition

Goal

To improve lexical and semantic language abilities (i.e., vocabulary, word meanings, word relationships) to levels commensurate with chronological age and grade-level expectancies.

Objectives

1. Student will *identify, describe,* and *utilize* curricular vocabulary encountered in story books, nonfiction books, textbooks, etc. (target = approximately 10 to 15 new vocabulary items or concepts per story or thematic unit, for a total of approximately 30 to 45 new vocabulary items or concepts per 6-week grading period). Progress will be measured using the following rating scale: **0** = student has no idea what the word or concept means; cannot identify, describe, define, or utilize the item expressively in context; **1** = student has limited idea of what the word or concept means; may be able to identify, describe, define it (with prompting or cueing), but still cannot use the word or concept spontaneously and expressively in context (e.g., when retelling or discussing a story); **2** = student has a fully developed understanding of what the word or concept means (able to identify, describe, define it), beginning to be able to use it expressively in a limited fashion (with prompting or cueing); **3** = student has a fully developed understanding of what the word or concept means; can identify, describe, define, and utilize the word or concept correctly and spontaneously in context when retelling or discussing the story.
2. Student will demonstrate *context-based strategies* for acquiring new vocabulary words or meanings such as the following:
    a. Using picture clues to infer word meanings
    b. Using whole-sentence meaning (i.e., the rest of the sentence) to infer the meaning of individual words within the sentence (e.g., "Skip that word for now and read the rest of the sentence, and then we'll go back and figure out what that word means.")
    c. Using previously read material and background word or world knowledge to infer or predict the meaning of new words (e.g., "This book, *Heidi*, is about a girl who lived in the Swiss *Alps*. Look at the picture, and tell me what you think *alps* are. That's right, alps are a type of mountain. What do you already know about mountains?")
    d. Using phoneme or grapheme cues to infer meaning of a new word (e.g., from the story *Heidi*: "That word begins with the letter *H,* and it tells you the *name* of the girl in this book. What girl's names do you know that start with *H* that make sense here?" or, "That word begins with the letters *c-h* and refers to the *type of food* that Heidi's grandfather made from goat's milk. What type of dairy product do you eat that comes from milk and starts with *ch*?")
        Rating scale: **0** = no mastery of skill; **1** = limited mastery of skill; **2** = complete mastery of skill.
3. Student will demonstrate *dictionary skills and formal strategies* for acquiring new vocabulary including the following:
    a. Ability to locate words in a dictionary using guide words and alphabetization skills
    b. Ability to use phonetic pronunciation key in a dictionary to pronounce words correctly
    c. Ability to identify usage and parts of speech using abbreviations in a dictionary entry
    d. Ability to read and understand definitions in a dictionary
    e. Ability to read and understand sample sentences in a dictionary entry
    f. Ability to subsequently define words without looking at the dictionary entry
    g. Ability to subsequently use words correctly in self-generated sentences without looking at the dictionary entry
    h. Ability to generalize new words and meanings to spontaneous classroom discourse
        Rating scale: **0** = no mastery of skill; **1** = limited mastery of skill; **2** = complete mastery of skill

of the word and the contexts in which it is encountered.

Even after children enter school, most new words are still learned from context, often while reading, especially after third to fourth grade. We have discovered that children's definitional abilities also follow a predictable developmental sequence and that children become better at deducing word meanings from context throughout the school years.

In terms of the type of instruction that is preferable for promoting lexical acquisition (in both normal and LLD children), it appears that a balanced approach that incorporates both reading and discussion of authentic literature (and thus exposure to novel words in context) along with some formal training in dictionary and definition-gleaning skills is warranted. Interactive vocabulary instruction like the kind discussed in this chapter appears to have reciprocal benefits. Specifically, instruction that focuses on vocabulary and new concepts enhances children's ability to infer meanings and improves their overall comprehension of what they read (Maclean, 2000; Rupley et al., 1999). Likewise, as their comprehension increases, so does children's ability to figure out the meaning of and learn new words from context (Maclean, 2000; Rupley et al., 1999). It is this kind of simultaneous top-down and bottom-up processing that contributes to the development of a rich, flexible, powerful lexicon in children.

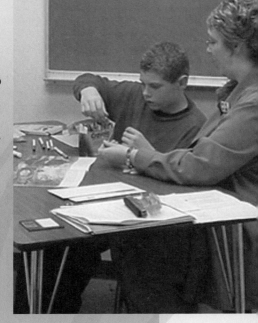

Chapter 6
Treating Spelling and Writing Deficits

Purposes

- Discuss development of writing and spelling skills.

- Explore the phonology-spelling link.

- Discover how to use invented-spelling techniques to help children produce closer approximations of conventional spelling.

- Develop strategies for improving language-learning–disabled children's written language content and form.

- Discuss how to help language-learning–disabled children plan, draft, proof, revise, and edit their writing (i.e., what good writers do) as they engage in meaningful writing experiences centered around thematic units.

- Discuss the speech-language pathologist's role in addressing handwriting.

Background

Although many speech-language pathologists (SLPs) have begun to incorporate aspects of written language and spelling into their intervention with school-age language-learning–disabled (LLD) students, some practitioners in the field still question why SLPs should intervene in these areas at all. SLPs may be reluctant to address writing or spelling skills because they feel these areas fall outside the traditional domain of oral language that they usually focus on with LLD children. To understand why SLPs can and should intervene in the area of writ-

ten language, we must first take into the account the growth in the number of children identified as LLD since the early 1990s. This growth, coupled with an increased understanding of the inextricable links between oral and written language, has resulted in a need for school-based SLPs to broaden their scope of practice (Butler, 1999a). It is becoming more accepted that the SLP's practice now extends to treating both spoken and written language deficits, often through collaborative partnerships with classroom teachers and other related service personnel in the school setting. Therefore, in addition to possessing broad knowledge about spoken-language development and disorders, the SLP must also become highly familiar with the linguistic characteristics of LLD writers in order to (1) analyze linguistic errors using samples from LLD writers' narrative and expository texts, (2) employ a variety of holistic and collaborative treatment techniques to improve written language in the LLD population, and (3) become adept at addressing both spoken- and written-language deficits during scaffolded reading and writing activities, using techniques such as authentic literature and thematically based art, drama, and play activities.

Many SLPs are surprised to discover that they already possess an abundance of prerequisite knowledge for working with LLD children's writing and spelling deficits. Their background knowledge in phonetics, phonology, semantics, syntax, and morphology is readily applicable to language in the written and the spoken modalities. That knowledge

Box 6-1 Common Characteristics of Problem Writers

Text and Sentence Level

- Production of shorter texts (fewer total number of words or total number of sentences)
- Less complex sentence structure
- Shorter clause length
- Omitted words
- Omitted punctuation (particularly lack of capitalization)
- Grammar errors, noun-verb agreement errors, tense errors
- Fragments and run-on sentences

Genre

- Difficulties with narrative genre (e.g., difficulties with pronominal referencing and narrator stance, omission of critical story grammar components—especially those dealing with characters' internal responses or plans or motives)
- Particular difficulty with expository genre (e.g., fewer lexical and grammatical cohesive ties; fewer logical adverbial clauses per sentence; overuse of sentence-initial *and*; less developed text structures; redundancies, abrupt terminations)

Semantics and Vocabulary

- Inappropriate word choice
- Restricted vocabulary (limited lexical variety)

Spelling

- Phonetic and nonphonetic errors, but nonphonetic errors predominate
- Word boundary difficulties
- Letter transpositions

Handwriting

- Faulty spacing between letters and words
- Mixed upper- and lower-case letters
- Mixed manuscript and cursive writing
- Messy, illegible handwriting
- Inconsistency

Modified from "Problem Writers: Nature, Assessment, and Intervention," by C. Scott, in A. Kamhi and H. Catts (Eds.), Reading Disabilities: A Developmental Language Perspective, *1989, San Diego, CA: College Hill; and "Learning to write," by C. Scott, in H. W. Catts and A. G. Kamhi (Eds.),* Language and Reading Disabilities *(pp. 224–258), 1999, Needham Heights, MA: Allyn & Bacon.*

must be augmented, however, by the wealth of information in the literature regarding linguistic characteristics of problem writers. Scott (1989, 1999) provides an excellent summary of common characteristics of problem writers (Box 6-1).

Additional characteristics of LLD writers that may be observed in the classroom or whenever they are asked to produce a written product include (1) reluctance to attempt spontaneous or independent writing tasks, preferring instead to copy written material from the board or worksheet (even if they don't comprehend or cannot read what they are copying); (2) failure to proof, revise, or edit during or on completion of a writing task; and (3) a tendency to focus more on correcting **mechanical errors** and creating a neater product than on improving content when they do revise their work (DeKemel & Ortego, 1994; Graham, 1997).

Development of Spelling and Writing Skills in Normal Children and the Phonics Versus Whole-Language Wars

It is estimated that an adult generally knows how to spell 10,000 to 20,000 words, yet in the spelling curricula (consisting primarily of words to be memorized from a weekly spelling list), children are explicitly taught approximately 3800 words during elementary school (Graham, Harris, & Loynachan, 1996; Scott, 2000). Accordingly there is some debate about how much spelling is taught and how much is *caught*, or learned spontaneously through natural immersion in literacy events (Scott, 2000). Scott notes that on the caught side of the debate, experts believe that children who are exposed to a literacy-rich environment will develop good spelling skills naturally as they engage in authentic reading and writing activities. Experts who espouse this view argue that too much direct, skills-based instruction, memorization, and drill in spelling is not only boring for students but also fails to achieve the desired result of transfer of spelling skill to text-level writing. On the other hand, researchers and practitioners who advocate the taught version of events are quick to point out that there is a paucity of empirical evidence to support more naturalistic spelling methods. Graham (1999) points out that even classroom teachers who support naturalistic

Box 6-2 Writing Development

Emergent Writing

(Ages 4 to 6 years)

- Children produce *draw-write combinations* or *multimedia productions* (i.e., children talk, draw, write, and dramatize the stories they are communicating).
- At first, writing may be only small part of the production (i.e., a few letters, letter-like forms, words).
- Later, proportion shifts such that longer text is accompanied by smaller pictures (pictures may be added after text is finished).
- Many children continue to draw small pictures on written work beyond mid-elementary school years.
- Children age 5 to 6 years may also write messages, labels, lists to help them remember and organize information.

Conventional Writing

(Early school years and beyond)

- Conventional writing is defined as the "ability to produce connected discourse that another literate person can read without too much difficulty and that the writer himself/herself can read" (Sulzby, 1996).
- The child understands sound-symbol relationships.
- The child understands words as stable, *memorable* units.
- The child understands that text is a stable, memorable object.
- The child is able to generate a written product within or across multiple genres (e.g., narrative, expository).

Modified from "A Sociocultural Perspective on Symbolic Development in Primary Grade Classrooms," by A. Dyson, in C. Daiute (Ed.), The Development of Literacy Through Social Interaction (pp. 25–40), 1993, San Francisco: Jossey-Bass; "Learning to Write," by C. Scott, in H. W. Catts and A. G. Kamhi (Eds.), Language and Reading Disabilities (pp. 224–258), 1999, Needham Heights, MA: Allyn & Bacon; and "Roles of Oral and Written Language as Children Approach Conventional Literacy," by E. Sulzby, in C. Pontecorvo, M. Orsolino, B. Burge, and L.B. Resnick (Eds.), Children's Early Text Construction (pp. 25–46), 1996, Mahway: NJ: Erlbaum.

Scott (1999) notes that during the last 2 decades, research in the area of writing development has switched from the *products* of writing toward the *process* of writing. Interest has been particularly manifested in the earliest stages of print literacy, leading examiners to study how writing emerges in naturalistic contexts such as home, preschool, and elementary school settings (Scott, 1999). Although writing had previously been construed as a late-developing linguistic skill based on a foundation of reading competence (Scott, 1999), it is now increasingly understood that the seeds of writing development are sown quite early. Indeed, writing is intertwined and emerges simultaneously with the development of the other linguistic modes such as speaking, listening, and reading. The various developmental stages of writing are summarized in Box 6-2.

According to the criteria stated in Sulzby's (1996) definition of *conventional writing* (see Box 6-2), most children could be classified as conventional writers by the end of first grade (Chapman, 1994). Many LLD children, however, reach mid- or upper-elementary school and beyond without attaining that important yet elusive status. Another essential element of being a conventional writer is *believing that you can write*. When asked, children still in the emergent stage often report that they cannot write, even though they can sometimes be persuaded to write something with coaxing (Scott, 1999).

Long-Term Outlook for Achieving Written-Language Proficiency in Language-Learning– Disabled Children

Unfortunately, the long-term outlook for achieving written-language proficiency in the LLD population is not very promising. Research indicates that the writing problems of LLD students do not disappear with age (Barenbaum, Newcomer, & Nodine, 1987; Montague, Maddux, and Dereshiwsky, 1990). Furthermore, the performance gap only widens with time (Newcomer and Barenbaum, 1991). Writing deficits in this population often persist into adulthood, even after improvements in spoken language and reading have occurred (Johnson, 1987). Given the importance of achieving writing proficiency in a literate society, it seems paramount that emphasis be placed on helping LLD students attain

or whole-language paradigms in theory nevertheless often continue to use direct instructional methods in their classrooms. This debate, often called the "phonics–versus–whole-language war," continues to rage in many educational and political circles. Fortunately, many researchers and practitioners are seeing the danger of letting the pendulum swing too far in either direction (i.e., a pure phonics or pure whole-language approach) and are recommending a reasonable, balanced curriculum that incorporates aspects of both instructional philosophies.

competency in the written modality as early as possible.

Difficulties in Writing

One plausible explanation for the difficulties LLD children experience in the written genre (and with language-based tasks in general) may be their failure to employ **metacognitive** and **self-regulatory** strategies (Graham & Harris, 1999, Singer & Bashir, 1999). Accordingly, the goal of therapeutic intervention with LLD writers would seem to be clear: to help them discover what good writers do before, during, and after writing, particularly when the purpose of writing is to summarize or respond to narrative and expository literature that they have read in school. Narrative writing in particular is considered crucial to the development of literacy (Anderson, 1978; Roth, 2000; Stein & Glenn, 1979), and the deficits displayed by LLD children in both narrative and expository written genres are increasingly receiving more attention in the literature (Roth, 2000; Scott & Windsor, 2000; Wong, 2000).

Plan-Write-Proof-Revise Method

In terms of helping the LLD child discover what good writers do, a coordinated intervention model known as the **plan-write-proof-revise** (PWPR) method meets the goal of addressing their self-regulatory difficulties and helps guide them through the **recursive** nature of the writing process. What follows is a series of therapeutic hints and techniques for utilizing the PWPR method to address written-language deficits in the LLD population.

Planning stage

1. Activate the LLD child's relevant background knowledge about the story or topic before any reading or writing activity by using a graphic organizer or another visual scaffold. Graphic organizers can be used (1) *before* reading to activate background knowledge, (2) *during* reading to keep track of facts and events, and (3) *after* reading to facilitate writing a summary, essay, or other written product. Examples of various kinds of graphic organizers include the following:
   - A *story map* is often used for fiction. This generally contains categories such as *characters, setting, initiating event, problem, attempts, consequences, resolution*, and *moral*.

   - A *fact map* is often used for nonfiction, or expository, texts. This contains categories such as *what I already know about the topic, what I want to find out about the topic*, and *what I learned about the topic*.
   - A *character map* explores items such as characters' physical and personality traits, motives.
   - A *timeline* is used for historical fiction or historical nonfiction.
   - A *comparison and contrast map* or outline can be useful for many types of expository texts and topics as well as for contrasting different fictional characters and their motives.
   - A *cause-and-effect map* or outline can also be useful.

   Many types of graphic organizers are now available commercially, and many school districts and teachers have preferred types of graphic organizers that they use on a regular basis with their students. For the sake of continuity, it is best to consult and collaborate with school personnel to determine the best type of graphic organizers to use with the LLD students on your caseload.
2. Discuss in advance what kind of writing assignment will be done on completion of the reading activity. For instance, will the written product be a paragraph summary, an essay, or a test with multiple-choice, fill-in-the-blank, true-or-false, or short-answer questions about the reading? Knowing ahead of time what kind of written product is expected helps to guide the reading process. The proficient reader knows what to look for while reading, always keeping in mind what will be expected on completion of the reading task.
3. Discuss the writing audience in advance (i.e., "Who will be reading my written product and what will that reader's expectations be?"). Some types of writing are more formal or informal than others, with the reader having differing expectations with regard to factors such as neatness or accuracy, depending on the assignment.

Writing-and-drafting stage

1. Emphasize that the first draft of the writing is just that: *a rough draft. Content* is the main focus of the first draft, not form and mechanics. Tell the child, "The purpose of the rough draft is to *get your ideas on paper.* Don't worry too

much about spelling and punctuation on the rough draft. If you can't spell a word perfectly, spell it the best you can for now, and then either circle or underline it. This will remind you that you need to work on the spelling while proofing and revising your next draft." LLD children often get stuck at the drafting stage. Because they can't spell (or don't believe they can spell well enough), they may not attempt to write at all or will write very little. Remember that *children learn to spell by writing*, not the other way around. Writing gives them a reason to improve their spelling, and they learn how to spell through the actual act of writing. Therefore, it is best to provide maximal scaffolding and encouragement to get them writing, even if it's just a sentence or two at first.

2. Provide various kinds of verbal scaffolding during their writing. Help them put their thoughts into words. Have them formulate out loud the sentence they want to write, then use a scaffolding technique such as **expansion** or **expatiation** (Norris & Hoffman, 1993) to add semantic and syntactical complexity, and then help them write the expanded sentence. For example:

> Clinician: *So let's think of a summary sentence to describe what happened on this page.*
> Child: *Jack got beans for the cow.*
> Clinician: *Yes, Jack traded the old cow for some magic beans. Let's write that sentence.*

3. LLD children often forget the sentence they have formulated before they can get it on paper. Have them use a **reauditorization technique** (i.e., saying the sentence over and over out loud after they formulate it) while they are transferring the sentence to the page. **Proofing-and-revising stage**

1. Emphasize that good writers often go through *multiple* PWPR cycles before achieving an acceptable written product (that's the *recursive* nature of the writing process).

2. After they have finished writing a sentence, have them go back and read it aloud to check to see if it sounds and looks right. Soon they will learn to do what proficient writers

do—that is, proof and correct their errors as they go along. Remind them to do the same thing at the end of each paragraph and at the end of the entire essay or written product.

Doing Plan-Write-Proof-Revise Method Out Loud

Eventually the LLD child may be able to perform the recursive acts of the writing process (i.e., written-sentence formulating, rereading, proofing, and revising processes) silently, but perhaps not for a long time. At first, the children appear to need to do these processes out loud. Perhaps difficulties with concept formulation, short-term memory, word retrieval, attention, and failures in their own silent auditory and rehearsal loop may be interfering with their ability to perform these processes silently. All these possibilities are certainly worthy of further investigation. In the meantime, it appears necessary and vital for some children to perform the processes out loud. Having the child perform the processes out loud during intervention also allows the SLP a window into the child's on-line processing (i.e., active processing) abilities. This in turn allows the SLP (through error analysis) to provide the child with additional scaffolding, modeling, cueing, and prompting as needed. Intervention too is a recursive process.

Again, be sure to have the LLD child focus primarily on formulating *content* on the first draft. Then with each successive draft the clinician and child can focus less on revising content and more and more on refining language *form*. It is important to note that *we never neglect written language form*. Factors such as correct grammar, spelling, punctuation, and legibility are extremely important for guaranteeing the clarity and acceptability of the written product to the reader. However, content must always precede form in the writing process. If there is paucity of content, form and surface features become somewhat irrelevant. It is helpful to think of this as a *pragmatic* issue: if the writer has little of interest or relevance to say and the writing has little content, it doesn't make much difference if commas and periods are in the right place, or if the handwriting is pretty.

How Many Drafts?

To achieve an acceptable written product, it takes as many drafts as it takes! The number of drafts varies according to many factors, including the skill level of the individual child, the goals of the assignment, the expectations of the reader, and the time allowed for the assignment. Many language experts believe it is more efficacious to spend additional time revising and refining a shorter piece of text than to have the child write a longer written product that has poor content and is full of form and mechanical errors. LLD children in particular seem to benefit and learn more from multiple revisions of a shorter written product.

Miscellaneous Hints

1. Emphasize to the LLD child that writing is a time-consuming, labor-intensive process but one that has great rewards.
2. Always remind the LLD child about *what the reader expects* in terms of content, legibility, clarity, and ease of reading. Written language has many formal rules, and the reader expects the writer to follow the rules.
3. Provide rewards (both intrinsic and extrinsic) for improving the written product. These may include the following:
   - Publishing students' work (e.g., typing it on a word processor)
   - Allowing children to illustrate and display their work only after it has been completely proofed, revised, and published
   - Sharing writing with others, including classmates; holding writing contests; consider team-teaching and peer tutoring; establish writing centers in the classroom—one table for drafting, one for proofing, one for publishing, one for illustrating (children cycle through the centers and help each other with the various steps in the writing process)
   - Writing for freebies (e.g., the class as a whole writes for free products or samples or coupons from retailers, manufacturers, and service representatives in the area)

Handwriting

Requirements for Handwriting

Handwriting (like writing in general) requires a complex integration of *cognitive*, *linguistic*, and *motor* capabilities. In the elementary school curriculum, handwriting is often included under the umbrella of writing *mechanics*. When it is broken down into its smallest elements, one can see that handwriting is a fine motor skill requiring mastery of the following:

- Proper grip of the writing implement (e.g., pen, pencil, crayon)
- Proper angle or alignment of the writing implement with the paper
- Coordination of intricate, continuous fine motor movements necessary for letter and word formation
- Eye-hand coordination
- Ability to maintain mental representation of the alphabetic letters while simultaneously transferring the symbol to paper (requires some use of short-term memory)
- Visual-spatial skills (left-right, top-bottom, directionality, spacing, size, proportion)

Role of the Speech-Language Pathologist

To understand the SLP's role in helping the LLD child with handwriting, the relationship between **legibility** and **intelligibility** must be understood. In spoken language, a child with multiple phonemic errors may be **unintelligible**. Phonological process, or minimal pair therapy, focuses on showing such a child that his or her sound errors result in a change in meaning (specifically, that his or her phonemic error productions result in the listener's receiving an erroneous message). A similar thing happens when a child's written alphabet letters are poorly formed or when the handwriting is very bad: the result is **illegibility** (again, the result is that receiver or reader cannot understand the message). As part of addressing overall written-language problems in this population, the SLP should focus on showing the child that poorly formed letters, incorrect spacing between words and letters, or anything that results in illegibility makes it difficult or impossible for the reader to understand the message. In other words, the SLP should emphasize that *writing* (just like speaking) is a *meaning-making process*, which can be negatively affected by the lack of clarity or incorrect production of the smallest elements (phonemes or graphemes) that make up the meaningful units (morphemes or words). However, if the handwriting problem appears to be primarily **motoric** (often accompanied by other soft neurological signs), a consultation with the occupational therapist and possibly the physical therapist is often in order.

Spelling With Intervention for Oral-Language Deficits

When attempting to justify why the SLP can and should be involved in spelling intervention, one can easily point out that spelling is, in essence, *written phonology.* The SLP, equipped with a wealth of background knowledge about the sound system of the language, is in an excellent position to work with the child on developing phonemic awareness, sound-symbol (i.e., phoneme-grapheme) relationships and the alphabetic principle, and sound segmentation and blending, as well as working on invented spelling when the child is unsure of the conventional spelling of a word. These activities are easily incorporated into a literature-based approach to intervention, which includes scaffolded dialogue during storybook reading and a variety of thematically related writing activities (e.g., creating graphic organizers and writing summary sentences, narrative summaries, character analyses, and responses to factual, interpretation, and inference questions about stories). During these writing activities, the SLP should urge the child to attempt to spell unknown words whenever possible. If the child cannot spell or refuses to try to spell the word, the following types of verbal scaffolding often prove helpful:

* "Spell the word as best you can for now; then later we'll come back to it and work on it some more."
* "Write the sounds you hear at the beginning, middle, and end of the word." (Note that many school-age LLD children will be able to fill in at least the *consonants* at the beginning and end of a consonant-vowel-consonant [CVC] word; *vowels* [i.e., the nucleus of the word or syllable] will usually be the most problematic.) For instance, the child who is attempting to write the word *reach* may able to write the initial *r* and the final *ch* with prompting and cueing (assuming the child has at least mastered phoneme-grapheme relationships for most consonant sounds).
* "If you're not sure about the middle sounds, leave a blank space for the sounds in the middle

and we'll go back and fill them in later." Keep saying the word out loud for the child (overexaggerating the sounds at the beginning, middle, and end) to help with this process.

* "Now let's fill in our vowels, or middle sounds. What are our vowel choices? *A, E, I, O, U,* and sometimes *Y* and *W,* right? Let's write those at the top of the page. Now, which of those vowels do you think goes in this space? Let's say the word again" (emphasizing the vowel sounds). Have the child write in his or her vowel choice, and then read the word with that vowel, even if it's incorrect (much as you would do during minimal pair or phonological process therapy, demonstrating for the child how the incorrect phoneme changes the meaning of the word). When the vowel is incorrect (for instance, if the child wrote *rich* instead of *reach*) the clinician might say, "Gee, you wrote the word *rich,* and that doesn't look or sound right. The word *rich* means to have a lot of money, and you are trying to write the word *reach* in your sentence, 'Jack wanted to *reach* the giant's castle.' What vowels are left to choose from that make sense here?" The clinician may also provide phonemic cueing such as "I hear a long-*e* sound in the middle of that word, and you chose the short-*i* sound, which is why the word says *rich* instead of *reach*. Which vowel or vowels should you choose instead to make the long-*e* sound in this word?" Point out that sometimes in English spelling you need two vowels to make the word *sound and look right* to the reader (e.g., *ea* in *reach*).

If the child responds with a phonetic spelling such as "reech," the clinician might say, "That's a very good phonetic spelling. You spelled the word like it sounds. But it's still not quite what the reader expects. There are some other ways to spell the long *e* sound. Let's think of some other words that rhyme with *reach*. Can you think of any?" The student probably will be able to, but if not, the clinician can assist by suggesting some, such as *each* and *teach*. The clinician can continue by saying, "Wow, look at that. In these words, the long *e* is made by using two vowels together, *ea*. It's the same in *reach*. Let's add *reach* to our long *e* spelled with *ea* list. Now we've detected a pattern of words that have the long *e* sound and are spelled with *ea*. We'll remember that next time." The clinician and child will refer back to the pattern in the child's Spelling Pattern Notebook when new *ea* pattern words are encountered (in order to add them to the list).

- Always put the target word back into its **meaningful context** after conventional spelling has been achieved. For instance, after the child has finally written the word correctly, the SLP should reread the sentence that the word was originally embedded in and emphasize the meaning (perhaps through paraphrasing, expansion, or expatiation). For example, "Yes, Jack was able to *reach* the giant's castle in the clouds because the beanstalk grew so tall." This reinforces the notion that spelling (and writing in general) is a purposeful, *meaning-making* activity.

Gradually, over time, participation in invented-spelling techniques similar to those just outlined during scaffolded thematic and literature-based writing activities will strengthen the child's phonemic awareness and understanding of phoneme-grapheme relationships, as well as increase his or her pattern recognition for regular and idiosyncratic spelling patterns in English. Perhaps more importantly, by participating in these sorts of activities, the child learns to integrate all aspects of language (form and content) to create meaningful wholes in the written mode.

However, invented spelling and other indirect instructional methods such as those outlined may be supplemented with a variety of other more direct, skills-oriented tasks as needed (e.g., phonemic awareness, word analysis, rhyming, sound blending, sound segmentation activities). Scott (2000) notes that some experts recommend a balance between direct and indirect methods of spelling instruction. Bourassa and Treiman (2001) also note that "from a practical standpoint, more extensive teaching may be required for some phoneme-grapheme correspondences than for others." Materials for direct instruction may be designed by the clinician for the individual child's needs; such materials are also readily available commercially. Whenever possible, direct activities should be tied to authentic activities. For example, if during an authentic writing activity a word with an idiosyncratic spelling pattern is encountered (such as the word *enough*, in which the

graphemes *gh* represent the phoneme /f/ and the graphemes *ou* represent the *schwa* vowel), the child and clinician might spend some time making a list of other words that follow the same spelling pattern (e.g., *rough, tough*). The original word and the words with a similar pattern might be entered as an integrated list in the child's spelling notebook. Later, when the original word is encountered again in print, the SLP can remind the child of where the word was first encountered and of the other words that display the similar pattern.

Dealing With Conventions of Print

Working in the written modality provides a marvelous opportunity to help children explore the conventions of print (e.g., punctuation and capitalization). Commas, periods, quotation marks, semicolons, and the like may hardly seem to provide a topic for scintillating conversation. However, when dealt with in the context of authentic reading and writing activities, we can, at least, make these print conventions seem useful and meaningful. Table 6-1 shows typical scaffolding techniques an SLP might use in the course of reading and writing activities to assist children in understanding some of the more common conventions of print.

The clinician would use some of the scaffolding techniques in Table 6-1 as follows. While the child is reading a text, if the child miscues by omitting punctuation (for instance, failing to pause at a period or comma), the clinician would immediately stop the child and say, "Oh, I think you missed something there—a piece of punctuation [pointing to the period, for example]. What is that piece of punctuation? That's right, a period [assuming the child correctly identifies the period]. Why do authors use periods? That's right, to signal the end of a complete thought [assuming that the child and clinician have discussed that print convention rule before]. So, what are we supposed to do with our voice to signal the end of the complete thought when we read aloud? That's right, pause, to give us, as readers, time to process the complete thought. So OK, read that part again, this time using the punctuation that the author provided."

Likewise, if the child is engaged in a writing activity (perhaps writing a paragraph summary of a story previously read) and the child and the clinician are in the proofing and revising stage, the interaction might proceed as in Box 6-3.

Table 6-1 Conventions of Print: Punctuation

PUNCTUATION	SCAFFOLDING TECHNIQUES
. (period)	*Question:* Why do authors use periods? *Answer:* To signal the end of a thought. *Question:* What should we do with our voice when we reach a period when reading aloud? *Answer:* Pause, to signal the end of the thought. *Answer:* Pausing also gives us time, as a reader, to think about what we have read so far, and to reflect on the meaning.

, (comma)	*Question:* Why do authors use commas?
	Answer: To separate words and phrases in series.
	    Example: Mary bought shoes, some hats, and a pair of gloves.
	Answer: To separate part of a sentence from another.
	    Example: After Mary went shopping, she met her friend for dinner at a restaurant.

! (exclamation point)	*Question:* Why do authors use exclamation points?
	Answer: After a sentence or character remark to show strong feeling or emotion
	    Example: He couldn't believe his eyes!
	Answer: Sometimes exclamations are used to show emotion for commands or *imperatives.*
	    Example: Mom said, "Clean up your room right now!"

; (semicolon)	*Question:* Why do authors use semicolons? *Answer:* To separate independent clauses not joined by a conjunction. *Example:* The road was long and narrow; the rain was blinding.
: (colon)	*Question:* Why do authors use colons? *Answer:* To start a list or to formally introduce a statement. *Example:* She found several treasures in the trunk in the attic: antique jewelry, old letters, and her grandmother's clothes.

' (apostrophe)	*Question:* Why do authors use apostrophes?
	Answer: To show a contraction.
	    Example: He can't find his car keys.
	Answer: To show possession
	    Example: This is Mary's piano.

" " (quotation marks)	*Question:* Why do authors use quotation marks?
	Answer: To indicate that a character in the text is speaking.
	    Example: "It's very windy outside," she commented.
	Answer: What's inside the quotation marks is what the character is saying. What's outside the quotation marks tell you which character is saying it.
	    Example: "Let's see a movie this afternoon," said Mary.

? (question mark)	*Question:* Why do authors use question marks? *Answer:* To indicate that there is a question or interrogative. *Example:* What time is it?

When the clinician uses these same scaffolding techniques again and again, consistently, the child should come to remember the conventions of print as they are used in the context of authentic reading and writing activities. This is likely to be a far more effective strategy than simply drilling children on the formal rules for print conventions such as punctuation, capitalization, and indenting. Children are more likely to understand and use a particular rule if they *see a purpose for it.* Likewise, the strategy of making the reading-writing activity a shared, meaning-making event places the burden on the communicative participants to use the various strategies effectively with one another. As in the previous example, emphasizing to the child that the child is the author and the child's failure to use punctuation effectively causes the reader to misunderstand the written message creates a *reason* to correct the punctuation error.

Box 6-3 Sample Scaffolded Dialogue During Writing Activity: Conventions of Print

---

Clinician: (Reads the student's paragraph aloud in order to proof and revise.) And then Jack climbed the beanstalk and then he went into the giant's castle he hid in the oven when the giant came in. (Clinician purposely reads the sentences fast and fails to pause at the point where the punctuation should have been.) Hmmm . . . did you notice anything funny about that? About the way I read it?

Student: Yeah, you read it kinda fast, and you didn't slow down or something.

Clinician: Yep, I think you're right. I think maybe you, the *author*, forgot to put in a piece of punctuation for me, the reader. After all, punctuation is what an author uses to signal the reader that it's time to stop, pause, take a breath, and reflect on what's been read. Look at this part. (Signals to what was just read.) Can you see anywhere in here where you, the author, gave me punctuation to signal the end of one thought and the beginning of another?

Student: (Laughs) No!

Clinician: Well, then how am I, the reader, supposed to know when to pause and reflect on the complete thought? I think you need to put a *period* in there somewhere! Where do you think one should go?

Student: Right here? (Points randomly at the text.)

Clinician: How should *I* know. *You're* the author!

Student: (Takes a little more care and rereads his own work aloud.) And then Jack climbed the beanstalk and then he went into the giant's castle. (Puts in the period this time, both with his voice and with his pencil.) He hid in the oven when the giant came in.

Clinician: Gee, that sounds much better this time! Let me *read* it and judge if as a reader, it *reads* much better and makes *sense* to me this time!

Miscellaneous Authentic Writing Activities for the Classroom and Speech-Therapy Room

The best practical advice I can offer the school-based SLP is to never miss a chance to involve LLD students in daily-living types of writing activities. By this I mean the kind of authentic writing activities that human beings engage in on a regular basis, such as labeling things, making to-do lists, writing lists of ingredients and instructions on how to do or make things, writing reminders on sticky notes (e.g., "I have a soccer game at 5:00 p.m. on Wednesday, November 25th"), writing directions for how to get to places, and writing reminders or informational notes to friends and family members. Are these not the very things that we adults use writing for on a regular basis? Then why not take every opportunity to involve children in these very same authentic literacy events as soon as possible? Here are just a few examples of how a school-based SLP or classroom teacher might make some of these suggestions a reality:

• Create a classroom post office (small cubbies or mail slots for each student, the teacher, SLP, etc.). I once had a teacher who even devised a mail system between her class and the class next door so those students could write notes and exchange with pen pals twice a day. Obviously, appropriate writing tools (e.g., notepaper, pens, pencils, envelopes) must be provided.

• Get one of the "cool" new label makers at an office supply store and allow students to help with organizing and labeling items such as supplies, drawers, cubbies, and shelves in the classroom or speech room. I borrowed this idea from an incredibly organized special-education teacher. Given that organizational skills are not known to be the strong suit of LLD children, this teacher was determined to make her classroom as organized and user-friendly for her students as possible. So she labeled each item such as shelf, drawer, desk, and box in her room with the strips from the label maker until she discovered that the students were as entranced with the label maker and the labeling process itself as they were with being able to locate items in the classroom! She began to use the label maker as part of her reward system, allowing students to use the label maker to label things in the classroom as reinforcement for good work, motivation, or attention. The catch, however, was that they had to use invented spelling and all their other strategies and techniques to achieve **conventional spelling** before they were finally allowed to key in the word on the label maker. It was amazing how hard the students would work to achieve conventional spelling in order to use the label maker!

- Ask students to help you make lists such as to-do lists or lists of items you need to purchase at the store (e.g., "I need to go to the discount store for school supplies this evening. Scott, would you help me by writing down this list of supplies that I dictate to you?"). Also, students can be asked to write down lists of ingredients for any cooking or food preparation that is done as part of thematic activities, and to make lists of steps for thematic art projects. For example, I often say, "Gee, I want to be able to remember the steps to this art project, in case I want to do it with another group. Angela, will you be our note taker today and record our steps for us?"
- Ask students who are capable of it to help you with logging and record keeping as part of your session. For example, "Whose turn is it to be in charge of the log book today? Aaron? OK. We finished reading on page 27 of the book *Heidi* and completed the *Attempts* section of our story map. Next time we will discuss the motives of the character *Heidi's grandfather* and continue with the *Consequences* section of the story map. We will also begin reading from a nonfiction book about the Alps. Can you jot down those notes for us in the log book, Aaron? I'll dictate while you write in the log book. Thanks!"

The point of these activities is to involve children in the kinds of genuine purposeful writing activities that we humans engage in on a regular basis. We can easily scaffold the activities in such a way that the child can participate at a level that he or she is capable of at the present time (and then gradually remove the scaffolding as the child becomes more proficient over time). My personal experience has been that students gain a great sense of pride and personal confidence from being involved in these types of activities. Through this involvement, they begin to view writing and literacy as part of daily routine living and not as some mysterious, difficult-to-master skill that is beyond their capabilities.

These are just a few practical suggestions for providing intervention for LLD children in the area of spelling and writing. SLPs seeking additional information and guidance in these areas should consult such excellent sources as Apel, Masterson,

Lombardino, Ahmed, Moats, Pollock, Templeton, and Bear (2000); Kamhi and Hinton (2000); Masterson and Apel (2000); Masterson and Crede (1999), Scott, (1999, 2000); Treiman and Bourassa (2000); and Westby and Clauser (1999).

Sample Individualized Education Plan Objectives

SLPs who are just beginning to address written language with their LLD clients often have questions about how to formulate appropriate goals and objectives for individualized education plans (IEPs). Box 6-4 shows some suggested objectives that reflect many of the abilities and techniques discussed in this chapter.

Box 6-4 Sample Individualized Education Plan Objectives for Writing

1. Student will engage in the following self-regulatory strategies during authentic writing activities:
   a. *Plan.* Create graphic organizers such as story maps, fact maps, and outlines to activate prior knowledge about topic, to guide reading, to keep track of factual information and events in stories and expository texts, and to facilitate drafting of written product.
   b. *Write.* Create successive drafts of items such as paragraph summaries, essays, and themes assigned by teacher and clinician on completion of reading activities, with attention to creation of pertinent and interesting *content* during first draft.
   c. *Proof and Revise.* Proof and revise successive drafts of items such as written summaries and paragraphs, with particular attention to revision of *form* on successive drafts (e.g., spelling, punctuation, capitalization, handwriting, grammar, and sentence structure).
2. Student will demonstrate improved phonemic awareness, sound blending, sound segmentation, and invented spelling abilities during authentic writing activities and structured tasks (e.g., rhyming games, word sorting, word segmenting, and word analysis).

Note: Progress on objectives listed will be measured through daily tallies of student performance, use of rating scales, rubrics, and portfolio assessment.

Measuring the Progress of Treatment

As mentioned in the IEP objectives in Box 6-4, students' progress in the area of written language can be measured using various kinds of quantitative and qualitative analyses. Many SLPs, teachers, and special educators have begun to use rating scales and various kinds of rubrics that reflect this kind of analysis. Figure 6-1 shows a writing rubric that I recently completed for use in measuring the LLD child's mastery of various writing and spelling self-regulatory strategies and abilities.

Summary

In this chapter we have seen that a balanced approach to spelling and writing instruction (i.e., one that incorporates a combination of authentic literature- and skills-based activities) is recommended for helping children discover the common patterns of English orthography. Many experts (Apel & Masterson, 2001; Bourassa & Treiman, 2001; Brown, Sinatra, & Wagstaff, 1996; Scott, 2000) now believe that important writing and spelling skills can be taught through **metalinguistic tasks** that allow the child to explore the *structure* of language (e.g., phonemic and morphological awareness, syllabification, segmentation, blending, rhyme, mastery of the alphabetic principle, and recognition of basic spelling patterns). It is now believed that early spelling development is largely guided by *linguistic factors* (Bourassa & Treiman, 2001) and that SLPs and other practitioners can engage in linguistic analysis of spelling errors to elucidate differences between children with normally developing language abilities and children with linguistically based spelling disabilities. Likewise, linguistic

---

WRITING RUBRIC

Student: _____   Date: _____

Examiner: _____

Rating Scale

4 = consistent, independent
3 = fairly consistent, needs some assistance
2 = inconsistent, needs assistance
1 = very inconsistent, needs maximal assistance

Plan

1. Creates graphic organizer (story map, fact map, etc.)	4	3	2	1
2. Activates prior background knowledge about topic	4	3	2	1
3. Uses graphic organizer during reading to keep track of facts/events	4	3	2	1
4. Considers reader's needs and purpose(s) of assignment when planning written product	4	3	2	1

Write/Draft

5. First draft focuses on content/organization	4	3	2	1
6. Attempts to spell unknown words (invented spelling)	4	3	2	1
7. Uses reference sources (dictionary, thesaurus, etc.) as needed	4	3	2	1
8. Uses graphic organizer to facilitate writing first draft	4	3	2	1

Proof/Revise

9. Proofs/revises for content/organization	4	3	2	1
10. Proofs/revises for form errors (capitalization, grammar, punctuation, handwriting, etc.)	4	3	2	1
11. Revises invented spellings to conventional spellings	4	3	2	1
12. Proofs independently without prompting/reminding	4	3	2	1

Total Score_____

Figure 6-1 Writing Rubric.

analysis of spelling and other types of writing errors is useful for remediation-targeting purposes.

We have also seen in this chapter that focusing on spelling for spelling's sake alone is not enough. Children must have a *purpose* for writing. They must understand that writing, like speaking, is a *meaning-making process*, the point of which is to convey a message. Anything that interferes with the successful transmission of that message (e.g., sloppy or illegible handwriting, a written message that contains sparse or disorganized content, or a written product that contains so many errors in form that the reader is distracted from the content) is problematic and must be addressed during the intervention process. We treat these problems as we would any other communicative breakdown—that is, by helping the child identify what caused the communicative breakdown, providing scaffolding or assistance on how to engage in message repair, and then acknowledging that the message has been received and understood. In other words, we treat the writing process as the meaning-making activity it is intended to be.

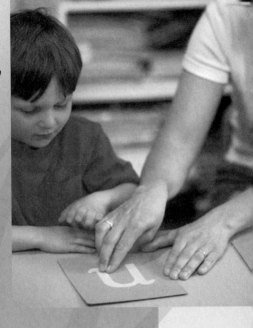

Chapter 7
Alternative Service–Delivery Models: The Move Toward Collaborative Consultation and Classroom-Based Intervention

Purposes

- Discuss trends that have led to the need for alternative service–delivery models in the field of speech-language pathology.

- Explore a variety of alternative service–delivery models including collaborative consultation and classroom-based intervention in its various forms (e.g., one teach–one drift, one teach–one observe, team-teaching).

- Provide suggestions for how to get started when making the transition to classroom-based intervention (e.g., how to approach teachers and administrators, how to select classroom-based intervention content, how to schedule and implement classroom-based intervention sessions).

- Describe how to troubleshoot problems that occur with classroom-based intervention (e.g., what if teachers leave the room during a classroom-based intervention session; what if the children in the classroom misbehave?).

- Describe how to document progress when using alternative service–delivery models, for classroom-based intervention sessions in particular.

- Discuss the importance of incorporating pragmatics into classroom-based intervention sessions (e.g., the cooperative principle, the politeness principle).

Numerous changes in the workplace (e.g., higher caseloads, educational laws, greater consumer involvement, increased requirements for accountability and cost-effectiveness) have led speech-language pathologists (SLPs) and other related service providers to explore **alternative service–delivery models** (ASDMs) for helping communicatively impaired children (Blosser & Kratcoski, 1997). These ASDMs include direct instead of indirect provision of services, consultation, collaboration, coteaching, inclusion, classroom-based services, team-based services, paraprofessional services, and a variety of other service options (Blosser & Kratcoski, 1997). Although emerging research suggests that these methods are becoming more popular (Beck & Dennis, 1997), there is still confusion about what is encompassed within each of these methods, how to choose the right method for each child, and how to make the transition from and integrate ASDMs with traditional service-delivery options. Additionally, the focus on new service-delivery models may have contributed to role confusion and questions of accountability for many SLPs (Prelock, 2000). Some SLPs have expressed concern that changes in service-delivery paradigms and a broadened scope of practice has forced them to become more like classroom teachers with a subsequent watering-down of speech-language therapy (Ehren, 2000).

This chapter explores the SLP's broadened scope of practice as it relates to ASDMs. Suggestions for how practicing SLPs can successfully employ a variety of ASDMs to help children with language disorders are provided. Classroom collaborative sessions and team-teaching using literature-based *communicative reading strategies* intervention as discussed in previous chapters is given particular attention, including how the SLP can modify these techniques for use in the classroom setting.

The Impetus for Alternative Service–Delivery Models

The Regular Education Initiative in 1986 urged special educators to provide more services in less restrictive, regular-education settings (Will, 1986). The Regular Education Initiative had an impact on the delivery of speech-language therapy services as well. Gradually, traditional pull-out therapy models (which are generally considered to constitute a more restrictive environment for the child) have come to be viewed in the literature as less optimal than classroom-based therapy approaches (Throneburg, Calvert, Sturm, Paramboukas, & Paul, 2000). Theoretical advantages of classroom- and collaborative-based approaches include (1) the SLPs' increased knowledge of curricular content; (2) teachers' increased knowledge of strategies for assisting communicatively impaired children; (3) SLPs' ability to serve a larger population, including at-risk students who might not otherwise qualify for speech-language therapy services; and (4) improved generalization of skills for the communicatively impaired child (Block, 1995; Cirrin and Penner, 1995; Ebert and Prelock, 1994; Miller, 1989; Nelson, 1989; Throneburg et al., 2000).

Unfortunately, research investigating the efficacy of classroom- and collaborative-based interventions has been sparse, and little is known about the number of SLPs who are actually employing these techniques successfully in school-based settings. Fortunately, several studies have begun to explore how SLPs are navigating the transition from traditional pull-out therapy to implementation of various ASDMs, including collaborative- and classroom-based intervention.

Beck and Dennis (1997) conducted a survey of school-based SLPs and teachers regarding their perceptions and opinions of various **classroom-based interventions** (CBIs). Survey respondents were asked to do the following:

1. Rate various factors that pertained to CBIs using a five-point scale (e.g., 1 = strongly disagree, 3 = neutral, 5 = strongly agree).
2. Cite advantages and disadvantages of various CBIs.
3. Rank various types of CBIs for frequency of use and appropriateness.

A total of 105 surveys were distributed to 75 teachers and 30 SLPs in three school districts (see Beck & Dennis, 1997, for further details). The overall response rate was 71%, with 54 teachers and 21 SLPs returning surveys. A total of 51 of the 54 teacher surveys were usable (i.e., returned complete), and all 21 of the SLP surveys were usable. The following categories (originally derived from a survey by Elksnin and Capilouto, 1994) were used to define the various types of CBI for rating purposes in the study:

- *One teach–one observe.* One team member (teacher or SLP) has primary responsibility for instruction while the other team member observes.
- *One teach–one drift.* One team member assumes primary responsibility for instruction while the other has responsibilities such as monitoring behavior and assisting students as needed.
- *Remedial teaching.* One team member instructs children who have mastered the material while the other team member instructs students who have not mastered the material.
- *Station teaching.* The material is divided into parts and each team member teaches his or her part to children at various stations in the

classroom; children are divided into groups that rotate among the stations.

- *Supplemental teaching.* One team member presents material in a standard way, while the other team member adapts or modifies the material for special-needs children.
- *Team-teaching.* Members of the team share responsibility for planning and presenting the material to students.

When responding to open-ended survey questions, respondents in the Beck and Dennis survey reported *advantages* of CBI such as the following:

- Clients remained in their natural school setting with more functional goals and did not miss out on classroom activities (57% of SLP respondents; 26% of teacher respondents).
- Peer modeling and improved social interactions occurred (43% of SLPs and 27% of teacher respondents).
- General student performance was enhanced, especially carryover of newly acquired skills (43% of SLPs).
- Communication between professionals was enhanced (29% of SLPs).
- The ability of teachers to help target and understand speech-language goals for clients was improved (24% of teachers).

Disadvantages of CBI cited by respondents included the following:

- Planning time was difficult to find (62% of SLPs; 31% of teachers).
- SLPs lacked the ability to target specific speech-language goals (43% of SLPs; 24% of teachers).
- There was a lack of teachers' support and/or lack of teachers' interest (33% of SLPs).

When asked to rate models of CBI as most or least appropriate, teachers and SLPs agreed that the team-teaching model was the most appropriate model. Supplemental teaching was ranked as second most appropriate by SLPs and third most appropriate by teachers. The one teach–one drift model was ranked third most appropriate by SLPs and second by teachers. Station teaching and remedial teaching were ranked fourth and fifth, respectively, by SLPs, and fifth and fourth, respectively, by

teachers. Both teachers and SLPs ranked the one teach–one observe model as least appropriate.

Interestingly, the model that was ranked as most frequently used by teachers and SLPs was the one teach–one drift model. The authors of the study speculated that although the respondents indicated that a team-teaching approach with shared responsibility was most desirable, a one teach–one drift model would be easier to prepare for, if, as respondents indicated, it was difficult to find time to plan lessons with other professionals.

The authors of the study indicated two major areas of concern resulting from the data collected. The first involved the number of negative responses given by both teachers and SLPs to the survey question, Have you had any training in classroom-based intervention? Only 12 of 21 SLPs and 13 of 51 teachers answered in the affirmative. The other area of concern was some SLPs' perception of a lack of interest or support from teachers for CBI. Beck and Dennis suggested the need for increased training of SLPs and teachers in the area of CBIs, particularly in the form of joint in-service workshops to establish collaborative goals and a greater sense of teamwork.

Hints and Suggestions

Having had personal experience with almost all the CBI models outlined in the Beck and Dennis article, I would like to add several personal comments and recommendations on how to get started and succeed with CBI. Perhaps the best way to accomplish this is by answering issues that SLPs have frequently brought up about CBI.

Getting Started With Classroom-Based Intervention

There are several ways to go about getting started with CBI. It is essential to obtain permission from school administrators first (specifically, the school principal or assistant principal, depending on which administrator tends to be more involved with day-to-day school operations and is more in tune with the special-education population in the school). This is particularly important if the administrator is not familiar with CBI, or if previous SLPs in that school have not used ASDMs before. It is best to start the process by giving the administrator a friendly note in his or her mailbox (to be followed up with a person-to-person meeting

To: _____ (Principal/Assistant Principal)

From: _____ (Speech-Language Pathologist)

Date: _____

RE: Request Permission to Implement Classroom-Based Speech-Language Therapy Sessions

Dear _____ (Principal/Assistant Principal),

    There has been a recent trend in the field of speech-language pathology to explore the use of **Alternative Service–Delivery Models** (ASDMs) with our students who receive speech-language therapy. These ASDMs include alternatives to traditional pull-out speech-language therapy, such as **collaborative consultation** (CC), where the classroom teacher and speech-language pathologist (SLP) work together to establish joint communication goals/objectives and intervention strategies for the child, as well as **classroom-based intervention** (CBI) where the SLP and classroom teacher actually plan and team-teach language and communication-based lessons in the child's classroom. These ASDMs may take the place of traditional therapy sessions, but more often they are used **in conjunction with** traditional, direct, pull-out speech-language therapy. Research indicates that advantages to CBI include children remaining in their natural classroom environment where more functional communication goals can be addressed; also, children do not miss out on regular classroom activities. Studies also suggest that CBI results in improved social interactions and better carryover of newly acquired communication skills.

    I would like your permission to approach certain faculty members about the possibility of implementing some CBI sessions at this school as an adjunct and supplement to existing pull-out speech-language therapy sessions. I would be happy to talk with you further about what is typically covered during CBI sessions, as well as to provide you with literature substantiating the benefits of this type of intervention, and its growing credibility and acceptance in the field of speech-language pathology. I look forward to being part of a collaborative team with you and the faculty and the parents of _____ school as we work together to address the academic and communicative needs of our students.

Sincerely,

_____

Speech-Language Pathologist

Figure 7-1 Sample Letter to School Administrator.

later). The letter might take the format shown in Figure 7-1.

A similar letter can be crafted to give to prospective teachers with whom you are interested in collaborating (Figure 7-2). I don't generally give the teachers the letter ahead of time, though; I usually find a moment to meet with them in person (e.g., in the teachers' lounge during lunch, or during their planning period) so that I can informally chat and explain the concept of CBI. I then give them the letter at the end of our chat as a follow-up. I also don't press them to make a decision about whether they want to participate in CBI right then and there. I ask them to get back to me later and let me know if they're interested.

It is also useful to use the terminology from Elksnin and Capilouto and Beck and Dennis (e.g., team-teaching, one teach–one drift) when explaining the various models of CBI to teachers and administrators, particularly when giving in-service training at faculty meetings (another important marketing tool, by the way, when you want to make the transition to ASDMs and CBI). I find that concepts such as team-teaching and one teach–one drift are readily understood by teachers when properly explained, and it is tremendously reassuring to teachers to discover that you plan to start with the one teach–one drift model or the one teach–one observe model in your CBI sessions. It is the thought that you might be planning to heap yet *more* work on them that turns most teachers off to the idea of CBI. Once they see CBI in action, most teachers are interested, excited, intrigued, and more than eager to come on board.

You may also wish to invite your administrator to watch some of your CBI sessions (after you've gotten your feet wet and gained some confidence, of course). It has been my experience that most

To: _____ (Teacher)

From: _____ (Speech-Language Pathologist)

Date: _____

RE: Request Permission to Implement Classroom-Based Speech-Language Therapy Sessions

Dear _____ (Teacher)

There has been a recent trend in the field of speech-language pathology to explore the use of **Alternative Service–Delivery Models** (ASDMs) with our students who receive speech-language therapy. These ASDMs include alternatives to traditional pull-out speech-language therapy, such as **collaborative consultation** (CC), where the classroom teacher and speech-language pathologist (SLP) work together to establish joint communication goals/objectives and intervention strategies for the child, as well as **classroom-based intervention** (CBI) where the SLP and classroom teacher actually plan and "team-teach" language and communication-based lessons in the child's classroom. These ASDMs may take the place of traditional therapy sessions, but more often they are used **in conjunction with** traditional, direct, pull-out speech-language therapy. Research indicates that advantages to CBI include children remaining in their natural classroom environment where more functional communication goals can be addressed; also, children do not "miss out" on regular classroom activities. Studies also suggest that CBI results in improved social interactions and better carryover of newly acquired communication skills.

Given that you have several students in your classroom receiving speech-language therapy services, I would like to know if you would be interested in participating with me in some CBI sessions. The format I propose is as follows. I would continue to see the children for one traditional pull-out session once a week, but for their other session, I would like to come to your classroom and implement a **collaborative language-based session there**. Initially, this session would involve NO PREPLANNING OR EFFORT on your part. The session would take the form of what is known as "**One teach–one drift."** In other words, I would plan the language-based activity and implement it in the classroom. I would ask that you "drift" around the room to help maintain student attention, monitor classroom behavior, and perhaps assist any student(s) who might require extra help. You would be free to join in the teaching aspect of the lesson at any time, of course! However, you would also be free to just drift and observe until you felt comfortable joining in. In my experience, most teachers are ready to jump in and participate in the actual team-teaching and planning of the language-based lessons within just a few sessions.

I would be happy to talk with you further about what is typically covered during CBI sessions, as well as to provide you with literature substantiating the benefits of this type of intervention, and its growing credibility and acceptance in the field of speech-language pathology. I look forward to being part of a collaborative team with you as we work together to address the academic and communicative needs of our students.

Sincerely,

_____

Speech-Language Pathologist

Figure 7-2 Sample Teacher Letter.

administrators (if approached in a respectful manner and provided with sufficient background information) are eager to embrace new instructional and interventional techniques such as CBI, particularly if these methods are shown to be inclusionary and beneficial for special-needs children.

Selecting a Collaborating Teacher

There are many ways to select a teacher with whom to collaborate. Factors you may wish to consider include the following:

- Select a regular-education teacher who has one or more students with speech-language disorders in his or her homeroom classroom.
- Select a teacher who teaches reading or language arts (i.e., assuming that the grade levels are departmentalized by subject).
- Select a special-education teacher who has a high percentage of speech-language–impaired students in his or her classroom (e.g., a self-contained classroom for learning-disabled students or those with mild generic disabilities, a

classroom for severely language-disordered students, a classroom for preschool children with disabilities).

- Select a teacher who seems open-minded and interested in exploring innovative instructional techniques.
- Select a teacher with whom you have a good working relationship (perhaps you have collaborated or worked well together in the past).

The point is that you should select a teacher with whom you have a high probability of succeeding in achieving a productive collaborative relationship. This is particularly important if this is your first venture into the world of CBI. Later, as you gain confidence and experience, you may wish to branch out and approach teachers who are less enthusiastic or who are a little more reluctant to experiment with CBI. You will also find that word of mouth is the best marketing tool available; teachers with whom you experience successful collaborative relationships will quickly spread the word to their peers, and soon you will find yourself being approached by other teachers eager to have you in their classrooms as well.

As a word of caution, I recommend that you initially perform CBI sessions with no more than one to three teachers in your school, particularly if you are in a large school and have a large caseload to manage. Do not let yourself become overwhelmed! The amount of planning and the logistical challenges of scheduling CBI sessions can be rather daunting, and it is better to strive for *quality* rather than *quantity*.

Selecting an Appropriate Classroom-Based Intervention Model

The type of CBI model should be dictated primarily by the students' needs, goals, and objectives, as well as the content and focus of the lesson. Bear in mind that it is possible and perfectly acceptable to switch back and forth between different CBI models as needed and to combine features of several different models within the same session or classroom. For instance, I have often found station teaching to be extremely useful for conducting writing activities in fourth- and fifth-grade language arts classrooms. During this kind of station teaching, the room is divided into stations (essentially tables or desks and chairs grouped together) that the chil-

dren cycle through as they complete the activity. For such a writing activity, there might be a planning station where children create outlines and graphic organizers of what they plan to write; a drafting and writing station where they actually write their paragraph summary or essay; an editing station where they assist each other with proofing and revising; and an illustration station where they create artwork and illustrations to accompany the text they have written. There may even be a publishing station where the teacher, the SLP, or a more advanced student uses the computer or word processor to publish some of the written work for display. Station teaching can even be combined with aspects of supplemental teaching and peer tutoring, so that language-impaired students get extra assistance with drafting, proofing, and revising their written product as needed. As can be seen from this example, the fact that CBI is versatile and flexible is an essential advantage to this type of intervention programming. Some of the greatest benefits of collaboration arise when the teacher and SLP brainstorm and experiment with different CBI models such as one teach–one drift or team-teaching for different lessons, tasks, and activities in order to determine which model works best, given different factors such as varied lesson objectives, curricular goals, student needs, and learning styles.

Scheduling Classroom-Based Intervention Sessions

There are many factors to take into consideration when scheduling CBI sessions, including the size of your caseload, the age and grade level of the speech-language–disordered students you service, and the type of speech-language disorders exhibited by the students. In other words, all the usual factors that contribute to scheduling decisions are still relevant. *Client needs should always take precedence in determining whether CBI is the most viable and valuable service-delivery option.* Assuming that a student appears to be a good candidate for CBI, the next dilemma is how to work CBI sessions into the SLP's already-busy schedule. The following are some useful hints, again based on my personal experience:

- Consider striving for a balance between traditional pull-out therapy sessions and CBI sessions, particularly if you are new to CBI. For example, if you are used to seeing your students in small groups, twice a week, consider making one of those weekly sessions a traditional pull-out session and the other a CBI session. This is a logical and natural way to make the transition into ASDMs and CBI. Also, the two service-delivery options (i.e., pull-out and CBI) often facilitate, enhance, and complement one other in various ways such as the following:

1. The SLP may witness communicative difficulties in the classroom that were not apparent during pull-out sessions (problems with formal classroom discourse for example).
2. The SLP will have the opportunity in the classroom to assess and reinforce carryover of communicative skills that have been addressed during pull-out sessions.
3. The SLP will still be able to deal directly with skills in small group or individual pull-out therapy that might not be as easy to deal with in a large classroom setting (in other words, the lower pupil/teacher ratio during a pull-out session will always be advantageous for working on some skills more directly).

In other words, maintaining a balance between traditional pull-out therapy and CBI has the potential to provide a best-of-both-worlds intervention program that is productive and appealing to all concerned. Also, a balanced approach—that is, one pull-out session along with one CBI session per week—may serve to calm the fears of parents, teachers, administrators, and even SLPs who are still uncomfortable with the thought of giving up traditional skills-based therapy and may be viewed as a reasonable compromise by those previously mentioned who fear the watering down of speech-language therapy.

- Strive for balance in terms of days of the week and times, to make scheduling easier and more consistent for all concerned (e.g., perhaps schedule sessions on Monday and Wednesday from 10 to 10:30 a.m., with Monday the pull-out session and Wednesday the CBI session, to maintain consistency and continuity and avoid conflicts with other related service personnel).
- Consider alternative blocks of time, if half-hour sessions are too short or constrictive for CBI

sessions. For instance, I have found that a half-hour session is often insufficient for a CBI session (in a classroom setting with many more students, if you only have 30 minutes, time seems to run out just as you are getting to the good part of the lesson). Therefore, if your schedule does not allow you to maintain both types of sessions and you, the teacher, the parent, the child, and other team members conclude that the CBI session is more valuable, you may wish to either (1) consider seeing the child or children in question once a week for 40 to 45 minutes in a CBI session and shorten the pull-out session to 15 to 20 minutes or (2) increase the length of the CBI session to 50 to 60 minutes and dispense with the pull-out session altogether. Again, the point is to think outside the box with respect to time limits for therapy sessions. Just because SLPs have traditionally seen children for 30 minutes twice a week does not mean they must continue to do so if alternative time parameters prove to be more effective. For example, witness the cycled treatment approaches advocated by some experts in the area of phonology, whereby children are seen for intensive, daily treatment for a period of several weeks or months. Perhaps it is time to become more freethinking and creative with scheduling in the language area as well! Some experts in the field have begun to argue that 1 hour per week of language therapy is ineffectual, and these children might be better served by short, intensive cycles of treatment administered daily over the course of weeks or months, followed by short periods of rest or break, followed by another intense period of treatment, and so on. Again, determining what time frame constitutes the most efficacious form of therapy for language-impaired children (i.e., how many times per week, for how many minutes, over how many months or years) has yet to be adequately addressed in the research literature. In the meantime, however, that should not stop practicing clinicians from being willing to employ ASDMs and break out of the traditional paradigm of twice a week for 30 minutes each session if, on a case-by-case basis, they judge that paradigm to not be in the best interest of their clients.

• Consider your *groupings* of children carefully. You can often maximize your scheduling and accomplish a great deal in a very efficient manner by thinking creatively and considering where children spend their day or part of their day. For instance, I once worked with a regular-education fourth-grade teacher who had four speech-impaired-only children (i.e., children enrolled in regular education, receiving speech-language therapy services for language disorders) in her homeroom classroom. Four children from one of the special-education self-contained classrooms for learning-disabled students were also mainstreamed into this teacher's regular-education classroom for art and music. Through careful planning and scheduling, the teacher and I arranged a collaborative classroom session once a week during the teacher's art and music period (i.e., when all eight of the children would be present in that teacher's classroom). Therefore, I was able to serve eight children from my 70-student caseload during that time period, and because the CBI sessions focused on literature-based intervention with accompanying thematic art, drama, and music activities, curricular goals and objectives from the teacher's lesson plan were successfully addressed as well. I also maintained the students' once-a-week pull-out sessions (small groups of three to four students each) in order to work on certain skills more directly, thus achieving the balanced intervention paradigm previously mentioned.

Working With the Collaborating Teacher

As previously stated, one reason teachers may be reluctant to attempt CBI is that they fear an increase in their already heavy workload. And who can blame them? The SLP can go a long way toward putting those fears to rest by assuring the teacher that he or she will not have to do much planning or even implementation of the classroom-based language lessons initially. I find that it is generally best to start with the one teach–one observe or one teach–one drift model of CBI, but others might have different preferences. After presenting the teacher with a letter similar to the one given to the administrator (and assuming the teacher has then indicated an interest in CBI), the SLP should follow up with another personal visit to communicate the following:

I'm so glad to hear you're interested in doing some collaborative language sessions with me in your classroom, and I'd really like to schedule a few sessions on a trial basis soon, to see what you think. If you like, we can do a one teach–one drift or one teach–one observe model, in which I plan and execute the lesson and you walk around the room and observe and also help me monitor the students' behavior and help maintain their attention to the task. How does that sound?

Usually the teachers are relieved to hear that the activity will not require considerable effort on their part, at least initially, and they are happy to have someone new come into the classroom, for the novelty factor if for nothing else! Most teachers are keen observers, however, and they will spend the first one or two CBI sessions doing just that: keenly observing your methods and how the students react. They tend to quickly catch on to the language-based nature of the activities, and often within just a few sessions they cannot resist jumping in and participating in the lesson. Before you know it, the one teach–one observe or one teach–one drift model has evolved naturally into a true team-teaching collaborative model.

Handling Behavior Problems

Many SLPs have confided to me that one of their main fears about CBI is going into a classroom of 25 to 30 children and having to deal with behavior management. After all, we generally only have to manage behavior in small groups, and that can be challenging enough! I urge SLPs to overcome their fears of behavior management. There are a variety of ways to manage behavior on a large scale, and the rewards can be tremendous. First, selecting the type of CBI model is important. The one teach–one drift model can be very useful for handling behavior problems during a CBI session. Generally the SLP can continue to lead the lesson while the teacher drifts and monitors classroom behavior, makes sure students are paying attention, provides one-on-one assistance to students, and performs other tasks as needed. Sometimes if students have a rowdy day, a temporary shift from a team-teaching model back to a one teach–one drift model for a session or two is all that is needed to reestablish order. Establishing a consistent system of rewards and reinforcement and other behavioral consequences is also useful. Usually it is best for the SLP to adopt whatever behavior-management system the teacher already has in place in his or her classroom and to apply that system consistently when in the classroom (e.g., students get their names put on the board for not attending or misbehaving and lose privileges such as recess or computer time if they get their names on the board). Applying the teacher's own behavior-management system consistently also establishes the SLP's authority with the students; students quickly come to view the SLP as a coteacher having equal power and status with the classroom teacher, and this often reduces or eliminates misbehavior and challenges to authority. It is often helpful for the classroom teacher to verbalize the SLP's authority as well, for example, "This is Mrs. X, and while she is in here, she has the same power and authority as I do. She can give out stars and rewards or withhold computer and recess time."

Handling Collaboration Problems

There are a variety of reasons why CBI might not work out for the parties concerned. Scheduling conflicts are among the primary reasons CBI sessions may become problematic. Children in special education are often receiving a variety of related services, not just speech-language therapy. Therefore multiple service providers have to coordinate their therapy times with the classroom teacher and with each other. Scheduling changes also tend to have a domino effect; in other words, if one service provider or the teacher changes the schedule, all service providers are affected. If, despite your best efforts, a CBI session has to be canceled because of scheduling changes beyond your control and a mutually acceptable alternate time cannot be arranged, you may simply have to return to a more traditional pull-out therapy format until scheduling conflicts can be resolved.

Another reason CBI may not be successful is lack of interest or participation from the teacher. On some occasions in my experience, teachers have viewed the CBI session as a chance to take a break by going to the teachers' lounge to make phone calls or grab a soft drink. Although this is certainly understandable if it happens on occasion, if it happens frequently or if the teacher is consistently elsewhere for most or all of your CBI sessions, then there is a serious problem. After all, it is impossible to collaborate and team-teach in the

truest sense of the word if your collaborative partner does not remain in the classroom. Sometimes this problem can be circumvented if there is a teaching assistant in the classroom who is interested in collaborating. Otherwise, it is best to be forthcoming and explain to the teacher that the purpose of the CBI is for the two of you to collaborate and team-teach, and if that is not going to happen, perhaps it would be best for you to return to a more traditional pull-out therapy format.

Protecting Your Voice

Don't forget to protect your voice! Keep in mind that when you are going into a classroom, you will be talking to (and above the voices of) as many as 25 to 30 other people. You will also have background noise (e.g., from the hall, the bell, the playground, the loudspeaker, air conditioner units) to contend with. Add to this the fact that you are talking all day during other CBI sessions and traditional pull-out sessions, and you have a recipe for developing a functional voice disorder. Fortunately there are now relatively inexpensive, portable amplifiers on the market that can be worn on the body with a lapel microphone that allow ample movement around the classroom while the teacher and SLP conduct the CBI session. Therefore practice good vocal hygiene and insist that your school district purchase these devices for you and your colleagues. In addition to protecting your own voices, you and the teacher will be setting a good example for the students by practicing good vocal hygiene (this is especially important for those students who may have voice disorders themselves).

Selecting the Content

The content and focus of the CBI session may take a variety of forms. However, it would be very logical to focus this type of session on what has come to be termed **formal classroom discourse**, or in assisting the language-learning–disabled (LLD) child in learning how to "do school."

Westby (1997) points out that, to be academically successful, children must learn how to do school. Learning to do school includes mastering *academic knowledge,* or the things to be learned, as well as *social knowledge,* or the ways of learning and getting along with others (Cook-Gumperz & Gumperz, 1982). Westby notes that the scripts for learning to do school are often *implicit* and can thus be particularly problematic for children with language or learning disabilities or those who come from culturally or linguistically diverse backgrounds.

Nelson (1989) describes learning to do school as a process whereby the child must navigate and master a variety of curricula, including the following:

- The **official curriculum**, or the actual course content that is to be taught at each grade level
- The **cultural curriculum**, or the world or background knowledge students must garner if they are to become functional, literate members of the society
- The **de facto curriculum**, which is based on the textbook, workbook, and other materials selected by the school or curriculum committee
- The **hidden curriculum**, consisting of teachers' expectations and criteria for determining who are the "good" and "bad" students in their classrooms
- The **underground curriculum,** comprising the rules for social interaction that guide peer interactions, perceptions, attitudes, and acceptance

Adding to the complexity of what children must master in these curricula are the various **social participation structures** of lessons in the classroom (Green, Weade, & Graham, 1988). These social participation structures include implicit rules about the following:

- Allocation of **communicative rights and obligations** among interactional partners (e.g., who can talk, where, when, with whom, how, and for what purposes during the lesson)
- **Gatekeeping** of access to people and information sources during the lesson (e.g., what is permissible to do if you don't understand or have a question during the lesson)
- Timing and sequencing of allowed interactions (e.g., waiting to be called on, answering in turn, not interrupting)

Cazden (1988) and Mehan (1979) reported that being able to understand and follow rules for directing attention, turn taking, and managing traditional **initiate, respond, evaluate** (IRE) exchanges constitute critical elements of the child's communicative

competence in the classroom. On the basis of these premises, one can begin to conceptualize the potential role of the SLP in helping the LLD child acquire these implicit rules about formal classroom discourse through the medium of CBI. Fortunately, a wealth of additional information has become available in recent years to assist the SLP in achieving that goal.

In a landmark study conducted by Sturm and Nelson (1997), quantitative and qualitative methods were used to analyze the specific discourse expectations of formal classroom lessons. Oral communication exchanges between regular-education teachers and their students in five classrooms each at first, third, and fifth grade (15 classrooms total) were analyzed across a variety of linguistic parameters of content, form, function, and complexity. These data, in conjunction with findings from prior research, were used to construct an information base for curriculum-based language intervention, in the form of generating *10 implicit rules* that students must infer to participate successfully in formal classroom discourse (Box 7-1).

Box 7-1 Ten Implicit Rules for Formal Classroom Discourse

1. Teachers do most of the talking and students do most of the listening, except when teachers grant students permission to talk.
2. Teachers give students cues or hints about when to listen closely.
3. Teachers convey information about content and procedures.
4. Teachers' talk becomes more complex in the upper grades.
5. Teachers ask questions and expect specific responses from students.
6. Teachers give hints or clues (often implicit) about what is correct and what is important or salient to them.
7. Students' talk should be brief and to the point.
8. Students ask few questions and should keep them brief.
9. Students talk to teachers, not to other students.
10. Students make very few unsolicited comments, and only about the process or content of the lesson.

Modified from "Formal Classroom Lesson: New Perspectives on a Familiar Discourse Event," by J. M. Sturm and N. W. Nelson, 1997, Language, Speech, and Hearing Services in Schools, 28, 255–273.

Other interesting findings from the study emerged, including the following: (1) teachers' talk showed increasing syntactic complexity with increasing grade levels and (2) turn-taking signals were more explicit in early grades and became more subtle or implicit as grade levels increased.

There is a wealth of other valuable information in the Sturm and Nelson article, but perhaps the most important information the reader gleans from their study is a clear understanding of the *implicit* nature of the rules for formal classroom discourse. In other words, these rules for formal classroom discourse are seldom *explicitly* taught; students are just supposed to know them and follow them. Students who are normal language learners are likely to pick up these rules spontaneously; this allows them to participate in whole-class discussions and formal lessons with little or no difficulty. LLD students, however, with their well-documented difficulties in areas such as processing implied information, interpreting nonverbal cues, and detecting what is salient are less likely to understand and master the subtleties of formal classroom discourse, and they may not be able to participate appropriately in the lessons. When students cannot participate appropriately in formal lessons, teachers may recognize that there is a problem, but they may inadvertently attribute these problems to *behavioral concerns* rather than to language-based communicative difficulties (Sturm & Nelson, 1997). It is the SLP's job to help the teacher understand the true underlying nature of these deficits and to assist in planning appropriate intervention strategies.

How then might an SLP translate data from the Sturm and Nelson study and others like it into designing and actually implementing a CBI session? First, it is useful to mention that there are some excellent programs on the market, such as Ellen Pritchard Dodge's *Communication Lab* (available from Singular Publishing) that may be used to address classroom discourse skills through a CBI format. The format and content of the *Communication Lab* allows the teacher, SLP, and students, through the use of various collaborative activities and role-playing activities, to identify what constitutes good communication and to practice and reinforce those communication skills in the natural environment of the classroom. For instance, the students, teacher, and SLP may target a specific pragmatic or communicative construct (e.g., turn taking, interrupting,

topic maintenance, eye contact, body language, tone of voice) and then do some role-playing that contains some form of communicative breakdown or failure by one or more of the participants. Then the role-players and classroom observers pause to analyze and discuss who was not a good communicator. Then the role-playing is redone, this time with the communication breakdown or error repaired, and the participants demonstrate good communication. Once again, the reenacted role-playing is followed by participant and audience discussion, this time with a focus on what constituted good communication and why.

Besides being fun and user-friendly, the *Communication Lab* is particularly beneficial in that once the general format has been put into place and the activities have been practiced during repeated CBI sessions, the original repertoire of activities and role-playing can easily be expanded to include almost any scenario the teacher and SLP deem necessary or appropriate. Additionally, the activities, because they focus on metaanalysis of communication skills, tend to result in the students, teacher, and SLP developing a shared vocabulary of communication during CBI sessions. Development of such a consistent shared vocabulary tends to make classroom discourse rules more explicit and leads to better carryover of communication skills, not just for the LLD children but for all children in the classroom.

Pragmatics

I hope that SLPs reading this text are seeing that all this discussion of classroom discourse rules clearly falls under the area of language known as **pragmatics**. Pragmatics is the area of language dealing with the effective social use of language. Again, there is a wealth of information in the literature to assist the SLP in addressing pragmatic issues. It has been my experience that many SLPs are unfamiliar with the groundbreaking work of H. P. Grice (1975, 1989), which is known as **the maxims** or **the cooperative principle**. Grice's work has tremendous implications for those wishing to understand the basic premises under which we operate in order to engage in successful communicative exchanges. These principles (when parsed and explained to children in language they can understand) can help make *explicit* the various *implicit* rules for conversation (Box 7-2).

Box 7-2 Principles for Being Cooperative and Collaborative in Conversation

1. Amount and sufficiency of information
   - Providing sufficient information to listener (i.e., not too much or too little)
   - Being sensitive to cues that listener *needs more information* in form of providing message repair, clarification, summarization, paraphrasing, or elaboration
   - Being sensitive to cues that listener *has had enough information* so that you can *stop talking*
2. Caliber, merit, and veracity of information
   - Avoiding misleading statements or blatant untruths
   - Backing up your statements with supporting evidence and facts
   - Supporting your opinions with information, including relevant background information, antecedent information, and contextual information
3. Organization and orderliness of information
   - Striving to be brief, concise, and succinct whenever possible
   - Avoiding ambiguity by saying what you mean in as clear a way as possible
   - Linking your ideas *temporally* and *causally* to achieve coherence and cohesion
   - Using your lexicon to chose best ways to express your intended meaning
   - Exhibiting variety and flexibility of word use to avoid sounding boring and stagnant, without being too flowery or overly descriptive
   - Avoiding rambling discourse that contains off-topic or tangentially related comments; avoiding giving nonsalient information; in general, observing the *less is more* or *economy of speech* principle
4. Pertinence, applicability, and suitability of information
   - Making your contribution to the conversation appropriate to *listeners, occasion, situation, time, place,* and *setting*
   - Taking into account all *contextual variables* when planning and structuring your discourse
   - Making judgments about listeners' level of *prior knowledge* about topic and structuring message accordingly (thus avoiding talking over people's heads or, conversely, being overly simplistic when listener is perfectly capable of handling more complex information)
   - Knowing when and how to *initiate, maintain,* and *switch* topics in effective, timely, and appropriate manner
   - Engaging in appropriate *verbal turn-taking* behavior (e.g., knowing when to take your turn in conversation, how to pick up thread of conversation when conversation is lagging, when and how to relinquish your turn, and how to gracefully invite and link others into conversation)

Others have built on Grice's work by adding to or revising the maxims. For instance, Lakoff (1973) condenses Grice's maxims to just two essential maxims:

1. Be clear.
2. Be polite.

Principle of Politeness

Leech (1983) (adapted by Fraser, 1990) developed the **principle of politeness,** which is stated as, "Other things being equal, *minimize* the expression of beliefs that are *unfavorable* to the hearer and at the same time (but less important) *maximize* the expression of beliefs *favorable* to the hearer." This can perhaps be further simplified to, "Tell people what they want to hear" (DeKemel, 2001).

The politeness principle adds six more maxims, including the following:

1. Tact (a keen sense of what to do or say in order to maintain good relationships with others or avoid giving offense)
2. Generosity (abundance in giving, kindness of spirit)
3. Approbation (the act of *approving* formally or officially)
4. Modesty (freedom from conceit or vanity)
5. Agreement (harmony of opinion, action, or character)
6. Sympathy (having common feelings; tendency to think alike; tendency to favor, support, or show concern for another's feelings or plight)

Using Information About the Cooperative Principle and the Politeness Principle

1. Clearly this information can be used for *conversational* or *discourse analysis*. SLPs can examine their clients' interactions with others such as peers, adults, and parents and ascertain where the students are having difficulty pragmatically. Chances are that SLPs will find *many* maxims within the cooperative and politeness principles that their LLD clients are violating, ignoring, or opting out of, or that they are simply unaware of in the first place. By definition, these pragmatic difficulties should and must be addressed during *social exchanges* such as small-group activities, whole-class interactions, pupil-teacher dialogue, and pupil-pupil dialogue.

2. Develop a **language of communication.** In other words, the SLP must educate clients about the *social aspects of language* and teach them the *purpose* of communication. The first rule I generally teach is that *language* (and communication in general) is a *tool* that people use to get things done—to accomplish things, transmit information, share and enjoy one another's company, and any tool can be refined and improved with practice. That is the essence of what we do when we come to speech class (or when I go into their classroom): we practice our communication tools and strategies so we can get better at it.

3. Using age-appropriate terminology, explicitly discuss with students *what good communicators do* (Box 7-3). The SLP can use Grice's maxims and the maxims from the politeness principle to *explicitly teach* pragmatic and communicative concepts such as approbation or tact. For instance, through role-playing and discussion during a CBI session, the group might explore various examples of being tactful versus not being tactful that they observe during a typical school day. Once they understand the pragmatic concept or principle in question, students often give concrete examples from their daily-living situations. Again, I recommend using Ellen Pritchard Dodge's *Communication Lab* for its role-playing suggestions as a starting point (you can use the role-playing scripts suggested in the

manual, or you can devise role-playing of your own using the *Communication Lab* format to illustrate situations in which people fail to adhere to the maxims, and then replay each scenario to illustrate how the participants could observe the politeness principles and how the communication proceeds much more smoothly as a result).

4. Be sure to explore what happens when people fail to adhere to the maxims (e.g., if someone rambled and failed to come to the point when the teacher asked him or her a question in class, or if the teacher asked a student to respond to a question and the student responded with a totally off-topic comment). Be sure to explore how the communication breaks down as a result in that situation, as well as how the student could then engage in message repair when the communicative breakdown has occurred. Point out that a person can almost *always* salvage the situation by engaging in message repair when communicative breakdown occurs. The trick is

---

Box 7-3 What Good Communicators Do

1. Take turns in conversation, invite others into the conversation, relinquish their turn to talk.
2. Make eye contact with others.
3. Use friendly body language and gestures.
4. Use friendly tone of voice—no sarcasm!
5. Express approval of other people's work.
6. Remember to thank others for helping them.
7. Remember to ask permission to borrow other people's belongings.
8. Provide enough information to the listener.
9. Repair their message when the listener doesn't understand them (repeat, rephrase, clarify).
10. Are good listeners as well as good speakers.
11. Are modest about their own success and avoid bragging.
12. Express sympathy when other people are hurting.
13. Stay on topic of conversation, switch topics when appropriate.
14. Consider how their words will affect others before they speak.
15. Keep their message organized (tell things in the order that they happened, focus on telling the most important things—leave out not-so important minor details).

Box 7-4 Rewarding Appropriate Pragmatic Behaviors When They Occur During a Session

Context and Participants. Students (third-graders) and speech-language pathologist are engaged in thematic art project related to the story *Jack and the Beanstalk.*

John (directed to student Heather): Heather, can I borrow the glue? I need to glue my leaves on the beanstalk. [*John displays appropriate turn-taking/requesting behavior.*]

Heather: (Hands glue to John.) All right. [*Heather honors John's turn-taking and request.*]

Clinician: John, I like how you politely asked Heather for the glue, instead of just grabbing it, and Heather, I'm pleased you honored his polite request. You guys used to just grab things from each other in here and get into arguments about it, but now you're observing the politeness principle, and things are a lot more pleasant with everyone sharing materials! [*Clinician contrasts previous inappropriate behaviors with current appropriate pragmatic behaviors and reinforces them.*]

(*A few minutes later in the activity.*)

Heather (directed to John): Wow, your beanstalk looks cool! How did you get the leaves to do that (referring to overlapping effect of the leaves)? [*Heather has just expressed approval or approbation of John's work, a maxim we had been discussing over the course of several weeks in therapy, i.e., the importance of complimenting others on their efforts.*]

John: I just stacked 'em one on top the other. You gotta put a little bit of glue just on the tip of each leaf but not too much. Want me to show you how? [*John has honored Heather's approbation and exhibited generosity by offering to help others.*]

Heather: Yeah!

Clinician: Heather, that was nice of you to compliment John on his artwork. His leaves really do overlap in a cool way! John, when you finish showing Heather how to make her leaves overlap, could you show the rest of us too? It's great how we're all cooperating and helping each other during this activity. [*Clinician labels and reinforces appropriate pragmatic behaviors.*]

---

to know how and be able to use the strategies for message repair (that is what you, the SLP, will be teaching and modeling during the session). So the goal of this type of pragmatic intervention (which can easily be implemented during CBI sessions) is to help students (1) identify the implicit pragmatic rules for communicating appropriately in particular situations, (2) avoid making pragmatic errors in those situations when possible, and (3) engage in successful message-repair strategies when pragmatic errors do occur (i.e., strategies that allow the communicative exchange to proceed successfully).

5. Remember, the SLP should not just focus on what the student is doing wrong. Focus should also be placed on what the student is doing right. This is a way of teaching to the student's strength and serves to reinforce and model good pragmatics (Boxes 7-4 and 7-5).

Over time, with repeated use of the same terminology (e.g., *be tactful, be approving and generous in your comments to others, repair your message, take a turn in the conversation, relinquish your turn, provide more information to the listener, be more succinct or to the point*), the children develop a lexicon of pragmatic vocabulary and pragmatic rules. The knowledge eventually becomes implicit—they will just know the rules, and the teacher and SLP can quickly correct children's classroom discourse problems with just a word or phrase. In fact, that is one of the most positive outcomes of this type of intervention in my experience. Classroom teachers are thrilled to discover a consistent lexicon and coordinated strategies for identifying and correcting these common classroom discourse problems (actually, these problems occur outside the classroom as well, but the classroom is where teachers encounter them and need help fixing them). The fact that SLPs have the knowledge to address these areas often comes as a delightful surprise to most teachers. Therefore, pragmatics is one of the areas we should consistently be addressing as part of the language arts curriculum (Box 7-6), and CBI sessions offer one of the most logical places to do it.

Box 7-5 How to Correct the Breaking or Flouting of a Maxim When It Occurs During a Session

Context and Participants. Classroom collaborative session, literature-based intervention (fifth-grade-age students, reading at approximately second- to third-grade level, enrolled in self-contained special-education classroom for language-learning–disabled students; total enrollment = 12 students.

Teacher and speech-language pathologist (SLP) are using the one teach–one drift collaborative model. Teacher is drifting around room to monitor behavior and assist students individually as needed. SLP is leading class in summary of previous session's reading (i.e., cover and first few pages of story *Heidi*) before beginning to cover new pages of text.

SLP: OK, who can summarize the information we discussed on the cover of the new story last time? Alvin? *(calls on student with raised hand).*

Alvin: It's about a girl who lived on a mountain with her grandfather.

SLP: That's right Alvin! And do you remember that last time we explored a new vocabulary word, the *name* of the specific mountains where she lived, in a country called Switzerland? The mountains started with the letter A—do you remember?

Alvin: (looks down.) No.

SLP: That's Ok. It's a new word. Does anyone else remember? Theresa? *(calls on an obviously eager student with her hand waving in the air.)*

Theresa (with smug tone of voice): The Alps. That's the name of the mountains. Alvin never remembers anything.

SLP: That's not true Theresa. First of all, Alvin *did* remember the answer to the first question. He remembered that the story was about a girl who lived in the mountains with her grandfather. [*Clinician challenges Theresa on her message inaccuracy—it is untrue that "Alvin never remembers anything".*] And second, remember when we talked about the politeness principles? Well, you just broke two of them. Do you know which ones? [*Clinician uses calm, even tone of voice during this exchange—focus is on pointing out which maxim(s) were broken, not on punishing the student.*]

Theresa: (Looking somewhat abashed now, shakes her head to indicate "No".)

SLP: Well there's the modesty principle for one, which says that we should not brag or be overly proud when we know the answer, because that makes other people feel bad. And the other is the tact principle, knowing what to say or not to say so that you don't hurt other people's feelings. When you said, "Alvin never knows the answers," you broke both of those good-talker rules. So what do you think you should tell Alvin now?"

Theresa (to Alvin): Sorry.

SLP: Thank you for apologizing to Alvin. Now, let's get out the globe again and see who can remember how to pinpoint and locate those Swiss Alps! [*SLP does not belabor the point—she simply points out which maxim(s) were broken, asks the student to engage in message repair (often a simple apology or rephrasing of a statement is all that is needed), and then moves on with the content of the discourse or interaction. The focus should be on correcting the miscommunication or repairing the communicative breakdown so that communication can proceed.*]

Measuring the Progress of Treatment in the Domain of Pragmatics

Measuring progress in the domain of pragmatics and formal classroom discourse can be difficult, because progress in these areas does not lend itself to traditional plus-or-minus or percentage types of scoring systems. By their very nature, abilities in these domains must be measured more descriptively, functionally, and holistically. The pragmatic rubric shown in Figure 7-3 is one example of how some of the maxims may be described and documented. The fact that these instruments are both qualitative and descriptive as well as quantitative to some extent (i.e., they do provide a score that can be documented and observed for change over time) is advantageous. (See Figure 8-2 for a similar rubric devoted to the documentation of formal classroom discourse rules.) SLPs are urged to use these rubrics as examples and templates for designing their own holistic rating scales and rubrics that will be appropriate for the populations they serve.

Box 7-6 Other Things That Speech-Language Pathologists and Teachers Can Say to Promote Pragmatic Awareness

Quantity Issues
- I didn't quite understand your message. Perhaps you need to give me more information.
- Thank you, I think I have enough information now.
- I think I understood part of your message, but could you clarify or elaborate a bit more for me?

Quality Issues
- Can you provide more evidence or background information to support your statement?
- Are you sure your statement is correct? Could you provide me with some additional evidence?
- Perhaps you need to check your facts one more time to be sure.

Relation Issues
- What you told me is not really relevant to our topic. Let's return to our topic, and you can tell me about _____ some other time.
- I'm not sure I have enough background information or knowledge to understand your message. Can you provide me with more background information or basic information about the topic first?
- I already have a fair understanding of this topic. Can you skip to the most important or more complex parts of your message to save time?
- We've exhausted this topic, I think. Why don't we move on to a new topic?
- We've completely explored this topic, don't you think? Let's move on.

Manner Issues
- You told me that in a kind of roundabout, rambling way. Can you be more specific or concise?
- The message you just gave me was kind of long and rambling. Can you tell me again, using fewer words and shorter sentences?
- As a listener, I am growing impatient for you to get to the point. Could you skip to the most important parts of your message?
- I think I lost your train of thought. Could you rephrase your message, making sure that all your points are in logical order?
- When you told me that story, I got a bit confused about the order in which things happened. Could you tell me again, and this time be sure to tell me what happened at the beginning, middle, and end, all in the correct order so I don't get confused?

Politeness Issues
- I think you may need to monitor your loudness or tone of voice and ask yourself if it is appropriate for this situation.
- Do you think that was a very kind or polite thing to say? No? Then perhaps you need to rephrase your message.
- Are you monitoring your body language? Sometimes our words say one thing, but our body language, gestures, and facial expressions say another.
- Let's remember to make pleasant words match pleasant expressions.
- Do you remember when we talked about what *being tactful* means? Well, ask yourself if that was a tactful question or comment, and perhaps then you need to rephrase.
- Remember when we talked about *bragging* comments versus *modest* comments? Well, that sounded like a bragging comment. Maybe you might want to rephrase.
- During our activity today, let's make it a point to take every opportunity to say generous, complimentary, and approving things to each other.

PRAGMATIC RUBRIC

Client Name: _____　　Date: _____

Examiner: _____

RATING SCALE
2 = Skill present or almost always present
1 = Skill intermittently present; skill emerging
0 = Skill absent or hardly ever present

AMOUNT AND SUFFICIENCY OF INFORMATION
_____Client provides sufficient information to listener (not too little; not too much).
_____Client is sensitive to cues that listener needs additional information (and thus provides message repair in form of clarification, paraphrasing, elaborating, etc.).
_____Client is sensitive to cues that listener has had too much/enough information (and thus ceases talking).

CALIBER, MERIT, AND VERACITY OF INFORMATION
_____Client does not say that which he/she knows to be false or untrue.
_____Client provides supporting evidence/facts to back up assertions, statements, and opinions.

ORGANIZATION AND ORDERLINESS OF INFORMATION
_____Client's utterances are clear, concise, orderly, succinct, and unambiguous.
_____Client links utterances and ideas temporally, causally, and logically (thus achieving coherence/cohesion).
_____Client uses his/her lexicon to choose best words to express intended meaning.
_____Client exhibits variety and flexibility of word usage (language is not flat, stale, or uninteresting).
_____Client avoids rambling discourse that contains off-topic comments, tangentially-related comments, or nonsalient information; in general, client observes the *less is more* or *economy of speech* principle.

PERTINENCE, APPLICABILITY, AND SUITABILITY OF INFORMATION
_____Client's contributions are relevant to the listener/audience, occasion/situation, time, place, and setting (i.e., *contextual variables* are taken into account when planning/structuring discourse).
_____Client makes judgments about the listener's/audience's *prior knowledge* about the topic and plans/structures message accordingly.
_____Client initiates, maintains, and switches *topics* in effective, appropriate, and timely manner (includes knowing which topics are off-limits in certain circles and judging which topics are likely to be welcome to certain listeners in certain situations).
_____Client engages in appropriate verbal *turn-taking* behaviors (e.g., knowing when and how to take his/her turn in conversation, how to "pick up the thread" or stimulate the conversation when it is lagging, how to link or invite others into conversation, and how to relinquish his/her conversational turn).

NONVERBAL
_____Client maintains appropriate facial affect during conversation (affect matches emotions and verbal message).
_____Client maintains eye contact during conversation (appropriate for cultural norms).
_____Client maintains appropriate spatial proximity to listener(s) during conversation (appropriate for cultural norms).
_____Client uses gestures in appropriate and natural manner to augment verbal message (appropriate for cultural norms).
_____Client uses appropriate prosodic features (rate, intonation, loudness, syllabic stress, pausing, etc.) to augment/enhance verbal message (or at least prosodic features do not interfere with transmission of verbal message).

_____**TOTAL POINTS**

Figure 7-3 Pragmatic Rubric.

Summary

In this chapter we have explored a variety of ASDMs, including collaborative consultation and CBI, for providing services to LLD children. We have also discussed how focusing on pragmatics (social use of language) and formal classroom discourse rules are natural content areas for CBI sessions. Suggestions for making the transition to CBI were provided (e.g., how to approach school administrators and teachers, how to plan and implement sessions), along with a review of various pragmatic principles such as Grice's maxims (the cooperative principle) and the politeness principle. Tactics for measuring progress in the area of pragmatics were also covered.

Chapter 8

Dealing With the Dismissal Dilemma and Long-Term Follow-Up of Language-Learning–Disabled Students

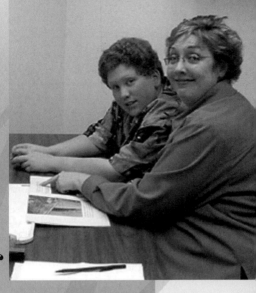

Purposes

- Discuss the dismissal dilemma with respect to LLD students.

- Review data with respect to the variables that speech-language pathologists generally use to determine if LLD children are ready for dismissal.

- Explore how speech-language pathologists can make better, more informed decisions with respect to dismissal, particularly given emerging evidence regarding long-term outcomes in LLD children.

- Discuss issues pertaining to follow-up of LLD children subsequent to dismissal.

Research suggests that children do not outgrow language disorders. Longitudinal studies indicate that many language-learning–disabled (LLD) children continue to exhibit problems in spoken and written language well into adolescence (Stothard, Snowling, Bishop, Chipchase & Kaplan, 1998) and even

adulthood. Accordingly, one of the most difficult questions that practicing speech-language pathologists (SLPs) face concerns *how long* a particular LLD child should remain in therapy, and *when* the child should be dismissed from therapy (Campbell & Bain, 1991). This chapter explores various aspects of what may be termed the **dismissal dilemma**, including the factors SLPs take into consideration when deciding to dismiss, and how follow-up subsequent to dismissal should be handled. I also discuss a pilot study I recently completed consisting of a survey of school-based SLPs regarding dismissal criteria and related issues.

The Dismissal Dilemma

Practicing SLPs face the question of when LLD children should be dismissed from therapy on a regular basis. Yet few research data exist to guide school-based SLPs in making this critical decision.

With the burgeoning focus on outcome measures and the need to document treatment efficacy in our profession as well as manage large and diverse caseloads, SLPs must have clearer guidelines to assist them in navigating the dismissal dilemma. Poor or uninformed decision making when handling dismissal may result in either a "life sentence" of language therapy for the child (Gantwerk, 1985)—that is, keeping the child in therapy long past the point when any true gains are being made—or in dismissal too soon, withholding intervention at times in a child's life when it might be most necessary and beneficial (Damico, 1988).

In general, one would assume that an LLD child should be dismissed from therapy when (1) the child has met predetermined language goals and objectives and/or (2) the child's performance has slowed or plateaued over a period of time (Campbell & Bain, 1991). Unfortunately, these assumptions ignore several larger questions such as the following:

1. Are LLD children ever truly remediated as a result of language intervention, and if so, how do we define and document that remediation (i.e., the *validity* issue)?
2. What specific criteria do SLPs use in determining when an LLD child is ready for dismissal from therapy, and what variables affect the decision-making process?
3. Are dismissal criteria similar across different school districts and different SLPs (i.e., the *reliability* issue)?
4. When are LLD children generally dismissed from therapy (e.g., after how many months or years) and what effect (if any) do factors such as age at the time of dismissal and the number of years in therapy have on long-term linguistic, academic, and job-related functioning?
5. If LLD children are not ever truly and completely remediated, how, why, and when do SLPs make the decision to dismiss them, given logistical issues such as time, scheduling, and funding?
6. What generally happens in terms of long-term follow-up and monitoring for the LLD child after dismissal? Specifically, are any mechanisms in place to assess their long-term functioning and to put them back into therapy if warranted?

Pilot Study

Method

In an attempt to answer some of these questions, I conducted a pilot study consisting of an open-ended survey designed to explore the issue of dismissal criteria for school-age LLD children (Figure 8-1). The survey was distributed to a group of public school SLPs (n = 100) in Jefferson Parish Public Schools (a suburban school district near New Orleans) and a group of SLPs (n = 15) in Lewisville Independent School District (a suburban school district near Dallas). Potential survey respondents were informed that participation in the survey was strictly voluntary and that confidentiality would be maintained. No names were used on the data-collection forms; however, for purposes of documentation and data tracking, the SLPs were asked to provide information concerning which grade levels they served and how long they had been practicing as school-based SLPs.

A total of 25 SLPs responded to the open-ended survey. On average, the SLPs had 12.86 years of experience (the subject with the most experience had 27 years; the subject with the least experience had 6 months). Some of the SLPs completed the survey form in its entirety; others only completed parts of the survey form.

Results

The principal investigator (PI) and two student assistants compiled the data. Because the survey format consisted primarily of open-ended questions, there was considerable variability in the nature and wording of responses from the participants. However, despite such differences in wording, there were marked similarities in the content of some of the responses, such that answers could in some cases be grouped into *content clusters*. I later provide samples of the most common survey responses for each question based on content clusters, followed by additional commentary added by some of the respondents. In an effort to ensure reliability, the two student assistants grouped the responses into content clusters first; both had to agree that a response fit before placing it into a cluster. The PI then examined any responses that the students disagreed about. If the PI agreed that a response belonged in a cluster, then it was placed

I understand that the return of my completed survey constitutes my informed consent to act as a subject in this research.

Survey on Dismissal Criteria for School-Age Language-Learning–Disabled Children

School District _____

Grades Serviced (K-5, 6-8, etc.) _____

Number of years experience as a school-based SLP_____

Date Form Completed _____

1. List **10 factors** or **criteria** you use to determine if the **school-age LLD** clients on your caseload are ready for dismissal. You do not need to rank order the items in terms of importance; simply list them as they occur to you.
    1.
    2.
    3.
    4.
    5.
    6.
    7.
    8.
    9.
    10.

2. List **5 specific language abilities** or **skills** (can be receptive, expressive, oral, or written modality) that you feel should be present in order for a school-age LLD child to be considered "ready" for dismissal.
    1.
    2.
    3.
    4.
    5.

3. Do you believe that LLD children are every truly "remediated" as a result of treatment/intervention?
   Circle one: Yes   No
   Comments on your answer:
   _____
   _____
   _____

4. Although "follow-up" on LLD children after they have been dismissed is not legally mandated, what, if any, formal or informal procedures do you think should be implemented with this population to ensure that they maintain levels of performance present upon dismissal?
   _____
   _____
   _____
   _____
   _____

5. In general, when you dismiss LLD children from your caseload, approximately how long have they been in therapy? (You may estimate here.)
   Circle one: Less than 1 year   1-3 years   3-5 years   Longer than 5 years

Figure 8-1 Dismissal Survey Form.

Continued

6. What kind(s) of research data would assist you in making more informed decisions about dismissal and follow-up of LLD children?

_____
_____
_____
_____
_____
_____

Additional Comments:

_____
_____
_____
_____

Please return the survey to:

Kathryn DeKemel, Ph.D., CCC-SLP
Assistant Clinical Professor
Dept. of Communication Sciences and Disorders
Texas Woman's University
P.O. Box 425737
Denton, TX 76204-5737
Phone: (940) 898-2474

Figure 8–1 Dismissal Survey Form Cont'd.

in the cluster (constituting agreement by two of three interexaminers). Responses that did not fit neatly into a content cluster, as judged by the PI and the assistants (i.e., agreement by fewer than two of three persons) were set aside and labeled *different* or *independent* responses and are not reported with the data shown later. Finally, the PI and student assistants compiled *summary statements* to represent each content cluster (efforts were made to choose wording that most represented and typified the various responses from that cluster). Following are the questions from the survey and the data and summary statement responses:

1. *List 10 factors or criteria you use to determine if the school-age LLD clients on your caseload are ready for dismissal. You do not need to rank order the items in terms of importance; simply list them as they occur to you.*

SLPs listed a variety of criteria they use to determine when LLD children are ready for dismissal (Box 8-1),

with "met all IEP goals/objectives," "plateauing or lack of progress over time," and "standardized test scores within normal limits" some of the most frequently cited reasons for dismissal.

2. *List 5 specific language abilities or skills (can be receptive, expressive, oral, or written modality) that you feel should be present in order for a school-age LLD child to be considered "ready" for dismissal.*

Again, there was considerable variability in the language abilities or skills that the SLP respondents felt should be present in order for LLD children to be considered ready for dismissal (Box 8-2). Some of the most frequently cited skills were *vocabulary*, *pragmatics*, and *reading abilities* at or near age or grade-level expectancies.

3. *Do you believe that LLD children are ever truly "remediated" as a result of treatment/intervention?*
   Circle one: Yes   No
   Comments: _____.

Box 8-1 Criteria Used by Speech-Language Pathologists to Determine If Language-Learning–Disabled Children Are Ready for Dismissal

- Student achieved all Individualized Education Plan goals and objectives.
- Student made significant progress in therapy; met maximal potential, based on what is realistically attainable for child.
- Student showed minimal or no progress over a period of time (i.e., *plateauing*). (Several respondents said "minimal or no progress over period of year.")
- Standardized testing revealed skills within normal limits (or "child no longer qualifies under state and local guidelines upon reevaluation").
- Amount of time student spent in therapy.
- Student Exhibits academic success without need of modifications by classroom teacher; language impairment no longer interferes with educational performance.
- Student Communicates successfully in classroom.
- There is evidence of carryover of language skills.
- Teachers no longer have any language or communication concerns.
- There is lack of cooperation or motivation or participation by student.
- Student has Frequent absences.
- Student has Frequent discipline problems.
- Parent reports satisfaction with language performance or feels child is ready to be dismissed (parental input).
- Student feels he or she no longer needs therapy, or child finds it is socially penalizing to remain in therapy (student input).
- Parent(s) requests dismissal because they feel attending speech-language therapy sessions is taking away time spent in classroom.
- Parent objects to dismissal (despite opinion of speech-language pathologist [SLP] that child is ready for dismissal).
- Nonstandardized assessment (e.g., language sampling, conversational skills) indicates student's language abilities are functional or within normal limits.
- Other programs or services provided at school will continue to reinforce language abilities.
- There is consideration of transition to middle or high school.
- Amount of home support/reinforcement supports dismissal decision.
- Other prognostic indicators (e.g., age, severity of disorder, presence of other disorders, socioeconomic status are a consideration).
- There is change in classification.
- Language age is commensurate with mental age.
- Social or pragmatic skills and ability to communicate successfully with parents, other students, teacher, peers supports dismissal decision.
- Student has ability to read at or near grade level.
- If caseload is too large, SLP determines which students are least likely to benefit from continued service.

SLP respondents disagreed on the question of whether LLD children are ever truly remediated as a result of language intervention or treatment, with eight respondents saying, "No"—that is, that they did not believe that LLD children are ever truly remediated as a result of treatment or intervention—nine respondents reporting, "Yes," and five respondents supplying mixed, ambiguous, or qualifying responses to the question (the remaining respondents did not respond to the question).

Sample "No" comments on question 3 were as follows:

- "LLD is a life-long disability. We teach children specific language structures, skills, and compensations but the core problem (difficulty processing and formulation of language) remains."
- "I feel LLD students will always be weak in the language area, but they can learn to compensate for these weaknesses as well as gain in these skill areas so that their weaknesses are not as apparent."

Sample "Yes" responses included the following:

- "Yes, if a student becomes an effective communicator despite delays and/or deficiencies."

- "Can be remediated to appropriate functional level."

Sample ambiguous or qualifying responses included the following:

- "I think this varies depending on the population and expectations."
- "Yes, within realistic expectations. If limitations are considered and modifications are employed, then these children can be given tools to function academically/environmentally. The important consideration is acceptance of the fact that some limitations may always remain."

- "It depends on whether language disorder is a primary or secondary impairment. Many students from nonstimulating, low socioeconomic backgrounds who enter school without basic concepts can be 'caught up.' Many others, because of primary exceptionalities (ex: LD) will always have difficulty."

4. *Although "follow-up" on LLD children after they have been dismissed is not legally mandated, what, if any, formal or informal procedures do you think should be implemented with this population to ensure that they maintain levels of performance present upon dismissal?*

Variable responses were also present with respect to the issue of follow-up subsequent to dismissal of LLD children from therapy. Some SLPs reported no formal procedures for follow-up, whereas others indicated that follow-up, when present, should be informal (Box 8-3). Some clearly felt that no follow-up was needed for LLD children after dismissal. Sample comments with respect to follow-up were as follows:

- "Follow-up should be in the form of being available as a consultant to parents/teachers to help with any future concerns."
- "I don't think we can guarantee follow-up—student could wind up being in and out of therapy all of school career."
- "Parents/families must be willing to do what is needed to help maintain progress; parents who are truly concerned with follow-up will call."
- "I do not feel there is a need for follow-up."

Table 8-1 Average Length of Time Language-Learning–Disabled Children Spend in Therapy, As Estimated by Speech-Language Pathologist Respondents

TIME IN THERAPY (YR.)	SLP RESPONDENTS REPORTING (NO.)
<1	0
1-3	4
3-5	11
>5	5
No response to item	5
TOTAL	25

SLP, Speech-language pathologist.

Box 8-4 Additional Research or Information Requested by Speech-Language Pathologist Respondents to Assist in Making More Informed Dismissal Decisions

- Specific checklist of minimal language skills (i.e., *minimal language competencies*) by age or grade level
- Predicted long-range outcomes (performance) of children with language disorders
- Long-term outcomes specific to students who receive therapy for multiple years versus those who receive therapy for shorter period of time (e.g., 1 year or less)
- Average length of time LLD children spend in therapy and how that relates to favorable outcomes.
- Typical areas of weakness or behaviors resistive to appreciable change even with therapy

5. *In general, when you dismiss LLD children from your caseload, approximately how long have they been in therapy? (You may estimate here.)*
   Circle one: Less than 1 year   1-3 years
   3-5 years   Longer than 5 years

Based on informal estimates by SLP respondents, LLD children appear to spend considerable time in therapy (Table 8-1) before dismissal. The majority of the SLP respondents (n = 11 of a total of 25 respondents) indicated that LLD students on their caseload spend approximately 3 to 5 years in therapy before being dismissed.

6. *What kind(s) of research data would assist you in making more informed decisions about dismissal and follow-up of LLD children?*

In general, SLPs indicated a need for additional information concerning minimal language competencies for children at specific age and grade levels, as well as information on reasonable expectations concerning long-term outcomes for LLD children (Box 8-4) to assist them in the dismissal decision-making process.

Conclusions

In general, the 25 SLPs who responded to the survey appeared to use a variety of factors when con-sidering whether an LLD child is ready for dismissal, with (1) "met all IEP goals/objectives," (2) "plateauing or lack of progress over time," and (3) "standardized test scores within normal limits" (or "Did not qualify upon re-evaluation") being some of the most commonly cited reasons for dismissal.

The SLPs listed a variety of specific language abilities they felt should be present at the time of dismissal, with age- or grade-level–appropriate vocabulary, pragmatics, and reading ability being some of the most frequently mentioned. Although no firm conclusions can be drawn at this time, it is tempting to speculate that these responses reflect a growing awareness on the part of SLPs concerning the intertwined nature of language and curricular content (also known as *language across the curriculum*). If so, then this is a promising sign that SLPs are growing accustomed to their expanded scope of practice.

It is also extremely pertinent that LLD children appear to spend multiple years in therapy (in some cases 3 to 5 years or more), according to informal estimates by SLPs who participated in the survey; Yet the SLP respondents did not necessarily agree on the question of whether LLD children can ever be truly remediated. Although no firm conclusions can be supported based on this limited sampling, it would seem to me that these findings reflect a certain amount of ambiguity and uncertainty on the part of SLPs—specifically, do we fear dismissing these children too soon because we are not sure about ultimate attainable outcomes (and thus we potentially keep these children on our caseloads long past the point that any true gains are being made)? Or does it just legitimately take that long (i.e., multiple years) to remediate a language disorder? It would seem essential that we conduct formal research to confirm exactly how long LLD children spend in therapy (on average) before being dismissed and to correlate that information with longitudinal studies and treatment efficacy and outcomes data. The question of how long it takes to remediate language disorders or to achieve acceptable, attainable outcomes has never been satisfactorily addressed.

This issue of follow-up subsequent to dismissal also deserves further attention, both as a research construct and as a practical one. Some SLP respondents appeared to feel there was no need for follow-up of any kind after dismissal, whereas others said that it is the responsibility of parents and teachers to monitor the language competence and communicative status of children in these cases. According to the results of this pilot study, when it does occur, most follow-up with LLD clients after dismissal appears to be informal (e.g., SLP consulting or conferring with classroom teachers). Given the strong emerging evidence that LLD children do not outgrow their difficulties and that language impairments affect the individual across the life span (Westby & Farmer, 2000), the issue of long-term follow-up and management of the LLD population is one we ignore at our peril.

Finally, results of the survey would seem to suggest that SLPs feel the need for more information about long-term outcomes of therapy in LLD children, as well as additional information on what may be termed *minimal language competencies* for students by age or grade level in order to make better dismissal decisions. Paucity of this type of information and the resulting lack of uniformity in applying dismissal standards no doubt leads to a variety of problems with reliability among clinicians, schools, school districts, and students.

Discussion

In terms of the strengths of this pilot study, the open-ended format of the survey did yield detailed, in-depth information from individual school-based SLPs regarding their views on dismissal criteria (specifically, the SLP respondents were not constrained by the format of the survey; they had the freedom to state their opinions and views explicitly). This detailed information will make it much easier to design a larger, controlled study in the future using a *close-ended* survey format (e.g., circle responses, rate criteria numerically). Such a close-ended format may also increase subjects' willingness to participate in the study, as the survey will likely not take as long to complete (several SLP respondents informally communicated to the PI that the open-ended format and length of time needed to complete the survey were deterrents to participation in the study).

In terms of weaknesses, the low return rate of the surveys and the resulting small sample size of SLPs completing the survey make generalization about these findings problematic. The open-ended survey format also resulted in a greater degree of variability in subjects' answers, making it difficult to quantify and directly compare responses across subjects.

Clinical Implications

Clearly, data from this pilot study and other anecdotal reports from school districts suggest that there are no uniform dismissal standards for LLD children, and although SLPs appear to be in general agreement on some of the factors for dismissal, they are unlikely to apply these criteria uniformly. SLPs are also clearly in need of more treatment efficacy and clinical outcomes data to guide them in the dismissal decision-making process, and the question of how to address follow-up subsequent to dismissal has not even begun to be adequately addressed. The issue of whether there should be standardized or uniform dismissal criteria and guidelines and minimal language competencies for LLD children will no doubt continue to be hotly debated in the field for some time to come. The advantages of establishing a set of minimal linguistic competencies and general dismissal guidelines for the school-age LLD population might include (1) ensuring better reliability across SLPs and school districts (thus preventing the possibility that a child could continue to receive services in one school district while being denied services in another based on arbitrary or unrealistic dismissal guidelines) and (2) allowing better monitoring of clinical productivity and long-term outcomes across service-delivery programs. However, there would certainly be distinct disadvantages to establishing and requiring adherence to such strict guidelines as well, including (1) failure to allow for flexibility when taking into account the *heterogeneity* of the LLD population and (2) failure to allow for the *variability* in caseloads across schools and school districts as well as a host of other logistical factors (e.g., socioeconomic, cultural, and linguistic diversity of students in the school or district, variations in school and district personnel, policy, and funding resources). Ultimately, the profession will probably have to strive for some sort of middle ground, consisting of establishing a set of suggested dismissal guidelines (I hope based on more clinical outcomes data and longitudinal research with the LLD population) while maintaining sufficiently open policies and flexibility for SLPs to continue to make informed dismissal decisions on a case-by-case basis.

How To Make Better Dismissal Decisions

In the meantime there are abundant resources available to assist SLPs in making more informed dismissal decisions. Much can be done with regard to the way progress on short- and long-term objectives is measured, how generalization of skills acquired during therapy is tracked, and how that information is then applied to the dismissal decision-making process (Campbell & Bain, 1991). In addition, the use of standardized test scores as the sole or primary criterion for determining dismissal needs to be revisited. As reflected in some of the responses from the survey in this pilot study, there continues to be a tendency to rely too heavily on results of standardized test scores when making dismissal decisions. The criterion for dismissal is often defined as "scoring no greater than 1 to 1.5 standard deviations below the mean on a standardized, norm-referenced language instrument" (Campbell & Bain, 1991). The language-impaired child is generally retested after an interval of time (perhaps

during a mandated 1- to 3-year reevaluation), and if he or she no longer qualifies according to district guidelines, the child is dismissed. There are numerous problems with this approach, including (1) well-documented issues concerning the reliability and validity of norm-referenced standardized test instruments and (2) the failure of such instruments to measure functional (i.e., pragmatic) communication abilities in natural contexts such as the classroom (Damico, 1985; Joffe & Doyle, 1996).

One possible solution to the problem of relying solely or primarily on standardized test scores when making dismissal decisions is to lobby administrators who set school district policy to allow for the inclusion of *criterion-referenced, holistic, qualitative, nonstandardized, informal assessment* procedures in the reevaluation process. This type of assessment may take the form of (1) language sampling and other types of discourse analysis, (2) teacher and parent interviews, (3) direct observations, (4) ratings of the child's success in classroom discourse, (5) academic grades in subjects such as reading and language arts, (6) portfolio assessment, and (7) anecdotal therapy data (e.g., daily logs, tallies, severity-rating scales). Inclusion of these types of assessment procedures ensures that a more complete picture of the child's functional communication abilities will emerge before dismissal decisions are made.

The issue of generalization (i.e., when the child will begin to show improvement without further direct intervention) is also closely linked to the dismissal dilemma and deserves further consideration. Clearly we do not want to dismiss an LLD child until we have some assurance that skills acquired in the therapy setting are transferring to other contexts, particularly the classroom. Generalization is notoriously difficult to measure and document, often because of logistical factors (i.e., the SLP cannot be everywhere with the child all the time). The SLP should keep in mind that generalization can also be measured through the type of holistic or qualitative assessment techniques previously mentioned (e.g., portfolio assessment, classroom observations, parent and teacher reporting, holistic rating scales). Therefore planning for the collection of this sort of data and making it easy and feasible to do so is an important part of the therapeutic process and an integral part of dismissal planning. Accordingly the SLP may wish to create a variety of items such as language-specific checklists, dismissal protocols, and tracking forms (Figure 8-2 shows an example of a dismissal protocol specific to formal classroom discourse) and to train parents, teachers, and related service providers to use these instruments well in advance of dismissal to ensure that the process goes smoothly.

Other Suggestions for Ensuring a Smooth Dismissal Process

It is always prudent to remind parents, teachers, and other related service providers before and at the time of dismissal that LLD students do not necessarily outgrow the need for language-focused instruction when they leave elementary school (Olivier, Hecker, Klucken, & Westby, 2000). Indeed, the LLD child is particularly vulnerable to communicative breakdown at times of critical transition and stress such as moving from elementary to middle school, middle to high school, and high school to college (and don't forget life transitions as well, such as moving to a new home or city, family trauma such as divorce or death in the family). Consultation with the school-based SLP or other service provider may be warranted if signs of regression in language and communication areas are observed during these times of transition. The SLP may also wish to educate parents and teachers about emerging evidence concerning the long-term effects of language-learning disabilities and apprise parents and students about community services that may be needed and are available in the future. For example, many parents are surprised to learn that "reasonable accommodations" in the form of preferential seating, additional time allotted for test-taking, and other forms of assistance deemed necessary and appropriate in the educational setting (based on the individual's disability and needs) are available through the Office of Disabilities and Accommodations on university campuses to assist adult LLD students who may qualify under Section 504 of the Rehabilitation Act of 1973 and the Americans with Disabilities Act of 1990. Increasing numbers of LLD students are participating in postsecondary education (Westby & Farmer, 2000), and language skills are deeply embedded in the high school and college curriculum and are predictive of academic success in those domains (Olivier et al., 2000). As part of our ever-changing scope of practice, SLPs need to be thinking ahead in terms of how we will help LLD students make the transition to postsecondary educational contexts, particularly because there is often little or no direct language intervention provided to them after they leave middle or elementary school. Often simply making parents and students aware that they will need to be assertive and proactive in seeking assistance and needed services across the life span is an exceedingly helpful first step in this process.

The SLP may also consider a variety of alternative service-delivery options when considering the needs of the LLD child before dismissal, given that *intervention* does not necessarily have to mean *direct intervention*. Indirect service-delivery options such as *tracking, collaboration,* and *consultation* may prove beneficial in moving a student toward dismissal (some may refer to this as a sort of *weaning-off* period), as well as helping to determine if the LLD child can sustain certain levels of performance without direct intervention before considering formal dismissal.

The SLP may also consider forming a dismissal task force or committee in the school or district to discuss crafting a set of suggested minimal linguistic competencies for each age or grade level. Committee members may include SLPs, special educators, language arts teachers, administrators, and researchers from nearby universities. These individuals have the expertise to take into account important variables such as curriculum, policy, culture, language differences, socioeconomic factors, developmental data, and recent research trends, which will in turn affect how minimal linguistic competency is defined for a given population in a given area. These suggested minimal linguistic competencies would be designed to serve *not* as rigid criteria for determining dismissal, but rather as an instructional data set to assist SLPs in managing the dismissal dilemma for their school-age LLD students.

Summary

In this chapter we have examined data obtained from my pilot study pertaining to dismissal criteria for school-age LLD students. We have discovered that school-based SLPs appear to consider a variety of factors when determining if LLD children are ready for dismissal, and that LLD children often spend considerable time (years, in fact) in therapy before dismissal. Often there appears to be little to

DISMISSAL PROTOCOL:
FORMAL CLASSROOM DISCOURSE

Student's Name: _____

Form Completed by: (circle one) classroom teacher, resource teacher, special education teacher, school psychologist, educational diagnostician, SLP, teacher assistant/aide, SLP assistant, other (please specify) _____

Name of Person Completing Form: _____

Date Form Completed: _____

Rating Scale
1 = Seldom/rarely
2 = Occasionally
3 = Frequently/often
4 = Almost always

_____Student answers questions readily when called upon (assuming student knows the answer), or student provides appropriate comment/statement to indicate that he/she does not know the answer when called upon.

_____Student provides sufficient information when answering questions/making statements in class (i.e., **quantity** of information).

_____Student provides information in clear, concise, succinct manner; avoids "rambling," unstructured discourse containing overabundance of fillers, mazes, false starts, revisions, etc.

_____Student **initiates** conversation with teacher and peers appropriately.

_____Student **maintains** conversation/discussion with teacher and peers appropriately (includes knowing when/how to invite others into the conversation/discussion; when/how to take a conversational turn and relinquish a conversational turn, avoiding off-topic and tangentially related comments, etc.).

_____Student knows how to **switch** conversational topics appropriately (includes knowing how to switch topics smoothly when topic of conversation has been exhausted, how to interrupt politely when necessary, etc.)

_____Student elaborates upon request, summarizes, repeats, rephrases, or engages in other message repair strategies as needed.

_____Student raises hand to request acknowledgment in order to ask/answer questions rather than blurting out questions/answers (or otherwise follows classroom rules for requesting attention/permission to speak).

_____Student follows oral directions and engages in metacognitive strategies when he/she fails to understand directions or otherwise needs assistance in carrying out task (e.g., raise hand to ask for assistance, ask a peer, etc.).

_____Student follows classroom rules about when to talk (e.g., only talks when it is allowed during certain tasks/activities, during breaks, etc.).

_____Student is adept at interpreting **nonverbal cues** from teacher that signal such things as "Listen," or "Time to finish your work," or "Stop talking."

_____Student displays appropriate nonverbal behaviors or body language in class (e.g., avoids mismatch between verbal message and body language, such as signaling defiance/noncompliance with body language while verbally acquiescing to teacher directives/commands).

_____Student uses appropriate rate, volume, and prosody (i.e., pitch, intonation, etc.) to support effective verbal communication in the classroom.

_____**Total Score**

Comments:

_____
_____
_____
_____
_____

Figure 8-2 Dismissal Protocol: Formal Classroom Discourse.

no follow-up of these students subsequent to dismissal, and no formal mechanism in place to assist them after they have been dismissed should they experience regression of skills during times of critical transition or as curricular demands increase over time. SLPs who responded to the pilot survey indicated they felt the need for additional information concerning (1) the predicted long-term outcomes of LLD students (particularly how the length of time spent in therapy relates to favorable outcomes for LLD children), (2) a specific checklist or minimal language competencies by age or grade level for LLD students, and (3) typical areas of weakness or behaviors resistive to appreciable change even with therapy in these children.

Given the emerging research evidence that children do not outgrow their language disorders and that these difficulties affect the individual across the life span, it seems critical that more attention be paid to the dismissal dilemma. SLPs must continue to weigh the host of variables related to dismissal very carefully, on a case-by-case basis, in order to make the most ethical and prudent decisions for our LLD students.

Appendix A
Sample Daily Lesson Plan

Client: Clinician:

Date:

Long-Term Goal: Student will improve receptive and expressive language abilities in oral and written modalities to levels approaching age- or grade-level expectancies.

OBJECTIVE	TEACHING STRATEGIES	MEDIA AND MATERIALS
1. The student will *read more fluently* and display *multiple strategies for decoding text* (e.g., use of graphophonemic cues ["sound it out"], use of context and picture clues, semantic clues) as measured formally and descriptively by measures such as clinician probes, oral-reading miscue analysis, rating scales, and teacher reporting.	1. The clinician will provide various prompts and scaffolding techniques (e.g., *Communicative Reading Strategies*, Norris, 1989) including preparatory sets, oral cloze, semantic cues, paraphrases, and expansions to help the student decode words and understand various levels of representation and meaning in the text.	1. Authentic literature (storybooks, expository texts) with clinician scaffolding as needed.
2. The student will improve *reading comprehension* as evidenced by the ability to answer *factual, interpretation,* and *inference questions* about stories and expository texts (target = 85% accuracy on comprehension questions over four consecutive probes). Progress is to be measured with the *question response rating scale* attached.*	2. See #1 under Teaching Strategies.	2. See #1 under Media and Materials.
3. The student will retell *narratives* in correct sequence and detail (with emphasis on temporality, causality, cohesion, and adherence to story grammar elements such as characters, setting, initiating event, problem, plans and attempts, consequence, resolution, moral). Progress is to be measured with the *holistic narrative rating scale* attached* (acceptable score = 17 or more of 20 obligatory points on the rating scale; target for mastery equals an acceptable score on four of six consecutive narrative probes).	3. The clinician will use graphic organizers (story maps, fact maps, character maps) to assist the student in learning story grammars and schemata and to improve the student's ability to retell narratives in correct sequence and detail. If the student's narrative retelling lacks sufficient detail or is lacking in factors such as causality and temporality, additional scaffolding will be provided by the clinician.	3. Paper, pencil, tape recorder, oral directions from the clinician to elicit narrative retelling.

Items noted as attached would be attached to the lesson plan.

Continued

OBJECTIVE	TEACHING STRATEGIES	MEDIA AND MATERIALS
4. The student will identify, explain the formal rule for, and use various *grammatical structures*, word formation and *sentence formation* rules (e.g., use of plural, possessive, third-person singular, past tense markers, compound words, contractions, adjectives, adverbs, rules for forming compound and complex sentences, and punctuation marks such as periods, question marks, quotations, and commas) during scaffolded reading and writing activities. Progress is to be measured formally and descriptively with the *grammar and morphosyntax rating scale* attached* and measures such as rubrics, portfolio assessment, and teacher reporting.	4. The clinician will target various grammatical structures, word formation and sentence formation rules during authentic reading and writing activities. The clinician will provide explanations, examples, and cues as needed to enhance the student's understanding of various morphosyntactical structures. Other activities (e.g., supplemental worksheets, grammar games) may be implemented to enhance the student's ability to carry over concepts to other instructional settings.	4. Authentic literature (storybooks, expository texts) and other material including a grammar rule guidebook, clinician-generated and/or published grammar worksheets from instructional teaching manuals, catalogues. Note: See the *skills and concepts to target (SCT) sheet* attached* for a list of specific morphosyntactical structures to be targeted for each story or expository text or thematic unit.
5. The student will identify, describe, and use new vocabulary and semantic concepts encountered in stories and expository texts. Progress is to be measured with the *vocabulary rating scale* attached (target = mastery of 10 to 20 new vocabulary items per concepts per story or book or thematic unit).	5. The clinician will target various novel concepts and vocabulary from fictional stories and expository texts and will use various scaffolding and cueing techniques to assist the student in learning various strategies for adding new words to his or her lexicon (e.g., using context to figure out word meanings, using dictionary skills, using the thesaurus).	5. Authentic literature (story books and expository texts), children's dictionary and thesaurus, other reference materials (e.g., globe, maps, atlas) as needed. See the SCT sheet attached* for specific vocabulary and semantic concepts to be targeted for each story or expository text or thematic unit.
6. The student will use *invented-spelling techniques* and other phonics and meaning-based strategies to spell new or unfamiliar words during structured writing activities. Progress is to be measured formally and descriptively with measures such as clinician probes, rubrics, portfolio assessment of the student's writing samples, and teacher reporting.	6. The clinician will engage the student in various authentic writing activities (based on literature and thematic activities), will urge the student to attempt invented spellings of target words, and will provide phonetic, phonemic, graphemic, semantic, and any other cues as needed to help the child ultimately achieve conventional spelling.	6. Items such as paper, pencil, dry-erase board.
7. The student will *write summary sentences* and *summary paragraphs* about materials read, using the *plan-write-proof-revise* (PWPR) metacognitive strategy. Progress is to be measured formally and descriptively with clinician probes and with the use of measures such as writing rubrics, portfolio	7. The clinician will engage the student in various authentic writing activities with a focus on mastering the recursive nature of the writing process (i.e., plan-write-proof-revise). The clinician will provide scaffolding and other assistance as needed, with the goal of helping the	7. Items such as paper and pencil.

*Items noted as attached would be attached to the lesson plan.

OBJECTIVE	TEACHING STRATEGIES	MEDIA AND MATERIALS

assessment of the student's writing samples, and teacher reporting.

student achieve as much independence in the writing process as possible, as well as increasing the student's understanding that writing is a meaning-making event.

8. The student will regularly engage in the following appropriate *pragmatic* behaviors during structured activities, formal classroom discourse, and conversations such as with peers or teachers:
   - Maintain eye contact.
   - Engage in message-repair strategies (e.g., repeat, rephrase, paraphrase) as needed and on request.
   - Provide sufficient information to the listener.
   - Ask relevant questions and request clarification as needed.
   - Enter into conversations willingly and spontaneously.
   - Initiate, maintain, and switch topics of conversation appropriately.
   - Use appropriate loudness and tone of voice for the situation or context.
   - Express approval of other students' work as appropriate during classroom situations.
   - Request permission (e.g., for classroom privileges, for borrowing of or use of materials) as appropriate in classroom situations.
   - Observe classroom rules for gaining the teacher's attention and answering questions (e.g., raise your hand, wait to be recognized before speaking).

Progress is to be measured formally and descriptively with clinician probes and teacher reporting. See the *pragmatic rubric* and *formal classroom discourse rubric* attached.*

8. The clinician will provide the student with conversational rules about what good speakers and listeners do to help the student understand basic pragmatic principles. The clinician will design various role-playing and other activities to help the student master these principles and will correct inappropriate pragmatic behaviors when they occur during structured activities and during conversation (e.g., during a narrative retelling activity, the clinician points out to the client that "I lost the main point of your message when you were retelling me the story. Could you tell me again, this time making your message more concise and to the point?" Or, "As a listener, I require more information to understand your message. Can you give me more facts and details?").

8. Conversation on various topics, and items such as tape recorder, dry-erase board for illustrating good talking rules.

Items noted as attached would be attached to the lesson plan.

Appendix B
Sample Speech-Language Evaluation Report

Client: Johnny Doe
DOB: _____
CA: 10 years

Clinician: _____
Date of Report: _____

I. Introduction

Ms. Jane Doe has expressed concern about the academic performance and language abilities of her son, Johnny Doe. Ms. Doe sought assistance from the _____ University Institute for Clinical Services and Applied Research in identifying any problems that may be interfering with Johnny's educational performance. Johnny is currently receiving a full psychoeducational test battery at the Institute to assess his overall academic and intellectual functioning. He was also referred to the _____ University Speech and Hearing Clinic for a speech-language evaluation as part of the multidisciplinary assessment.

II. Client Interview

According to an interview with Johnny, he enjoys attending school and is currently enrolled in fourth grade. His favorite subject is reading, and his least favorite is math. He enjoys playing computer games and has many friends.

III. Conversational Sample

During a brief conversational sample, Johnny displayed appropriate pragmatic abilities in the area of eye contact and willingness to engage in verbal interaction with the clinician. Johnny did have difficulty maintaining topics of conversation. He often switched topics inappropriately and made several tangential or off-topic remarks. There were also instances where he failed to provide sufficient information to the listener, requiring the listener to ask Johnny for more information or to engage in message repair. Johnny was able to repair his messages by repeating or paraphrasing, with prompting from the clinician.

IV. Oral Mechanism Examination

An oral mechanism examination revealed no apparent structural or functional abnormalities. A normal occlusion (i.e., bite pattern between upper and lower teeth/jaw) was noted. Johnny presented with normal diadochokinetic rates (i.e., ability to rapidly repeat syllables such as *puh puh puh*). No abnormalities in structure or function were noted when examining the tongue, lips, hard palate, soft palate, or palatopharyngeal mechanism. All structures/functions appeared normal and adequate for speech production purposes. Voice quality, fluency, and prosody (i.e., rate, pitch, inflection) also appeared within normal limits.

V. Administration of *Clinical Evaluation of Language Fundamentals—Third Edition* (CELF-3)

The following subtests of the CELF-3 were administered in order to obtain information about Johnny's expressive and receptive language abilities:

Subtest*	Standard Score
Concepts and Directions	12
Word Classes	10
Semantic Relationships	15
**Receptive Language Score	114

Continued

Formulated Sentences	4
Recalling Sentences	7
Sentence Assembly	9
Expressive Language Score**	**80**
Total Language Score**	**96**

*Mean for subtest standard scores is 10 with a standard deviation (SD) of ± 3.

**Mean for Composite Receptive and Expressive Language Scores and Total Language scores is 100 with a standard deviation (SD) of ± 15.

Results on the CELF–3 indicated receptive language abilities to be above average for chronological age expectancies (1 standard deviation about the mean). Johnny exhibited a mild overall delay in the area of expressive language abilities based on results of the CELF–3 (a score of slightly more than one standard deviation below the mean). However, analysis of individual subtest scores revealed a severe weakness in the ability to formulate sentences (score that was 2 standard deviations below the mean), along with a mild weakness in the ability to recall sentences (score 1 standard deviation below the mean). What is perhaps most significant about Johnny's scores on the CELF–3 is the noticeable gap between his receptive and expressive language abilities. This gap has both clinical and academic implications; he is likely to have difficulty expressing what he knows in the academic setting (particularly given his weakness in formulating sentences). Children who know more than they can express are likely to experience a good deal of frustration as well.

VI.   Narrative Sample

Johnny was asked to read aloud from a children's fiction story book (approximately late fourth-grade level). After the oral reading, he was instructed to "retell the story as if you were telling it to someone who has not read the story before." The transcribed narrative sample and narrative scoring form is attached to this document.

Johnny's narrative was rated using a narrative scoring criterion that is intended to evaluate adherence to story structure, inclusion of major plot episodes, and ability to present the narrative with temporality, causality, and coherence. Johnny scored 13 out of 20 possible obligatory points (i.e., points for obligatory elements that should be present in a narrative) on his narrative retelling. This is indicative of a "low average" narrative retelling based on this particular scoring system. This task appeared to be somewhat difficult for Johnny, and he required some prompting from the clinician to complete the task. It appeared that he possessed the macrostructure of the original story in his memory (i.e., the main plot elements) but was having significant difficulty putting those plot elements into his own words for the purpose of conveying his thoughts to others. His narrative retelling was characterized by absence of setting, statement of problem, plans to solve the problem, or resolution of the problem. His narrative also failed to establish appropriate causality (logical cause-effect relationships between characters, actions, and events) and displayed some incorrect usage of relational and transitional terms such as *so* and *but*. Johnny got somewhat stuck about halfway through the narrative retelling and paused and pointed out to the examiners, "This always happens to me." When asked to explain what he meant, Johnny stated that when he is attempting to remember information from a story or something that he has read, he often remembers "parts" but "not the whole thing," and has trouble "telling it back to the teacher." This would seem to substantiate information gleaned from formal testing (i.e., on the CELF–3, Johnny had difficulty with expressive subtests that required formulating sentences and sentence recall). Given that narratives (both the ability to comprehend and produce them) form a significant part of the language arts curriculum in elementary school, it is expected that Johnny's difficulty with the narrative genre would contribute to academic difficulty in the school setting.

Although a formal reading miscue analysis on Johnny's reading of the original story was not conducted (given that he was in the process of receiving a formal reading test battery by educational specialists at the Institute), informal data regarding his reading comprehension and word attack strategies was recorded to supplement data on his overall spoken and written language abilities. Johnny displayed many fluency-related miscues characterized by slow reading rate, word-by-word reading (i.e., reading with somewhat flat, monotone voice), frequent pauses, and revisions. Accuracy-related miscues (i.e., substitutions, omissions) were also present, and when they did occur, they were usually (but not always) self-corrected. The overall impression is that Johnny struggles with the form aspects of the print (i.e., the phoneme-grapheme, or sound-letter, relationships; the written grammar, or morphosyntactic, structure of sentences; punctuation, etc.). Struggles with these surface aspects of print no doubt make it difficult for him to access the deeper meaning of the text, particularly the implied, more inferential types of information (i.e., the information that the author does not come right out and say in the text but that strong readers are usually capable of picking up between the lines). The goal of working with Johnny in intervention should be to help him become a more balanced, strategic reader (i.e., one who is capable of utilizing multiple strategies for decoding and accessing the underlying meaning of the text).

VII. Parent Interview

After testing was completed, a parent interview was conducted with Ms. Doe to obtain her initial impressions of the testing data and to discuss possible intervention strategies for Johnny. Ms. Doe provided background on Johnny's speech-language history (he has a history of being a "late talker" and has been diagnosed with dyslexia in the past). Ms. Doe is eager for Johnny to get the assistance he needs to help him perform up to his potential in the academic setting. Ms. Doe too has noticed his difficulties with areas such as expressive language (particularly vocabulary and word-finding when he was younger—a problem that is still apparent on occasion today), the narrative genre, memory/recall, and word-attack skills, all of which were evident during the speech-language evaluation today.

VIII. Teacher Interview

A telephone interview with Ms. Smith, Johnny's teacher at _____ Elementary school, confirmed that Johnny is having considerable difficulty with certain aspects of the language arts curriculum. Mrs. Smith reported that Johnny gets easily frustrated during tasks that require him to remember and recite information from lessons and texts, and that, although she sometimes senses that he knows the answer, he appears to have difficulty putting his ideas into words. Ms. Smith indicated that Johnny becomes easily frustrated by these difficulties and often does not want to attempt or reattempt to answer questions in class, even when she provides extra help or assistance. Ms. Smith notices significant difficulty with Johnny's writing abilities; specifically, that it takes him "forever" to finish a writing assignment, and that he seldom if ever proofs or corrects his work before turning it in. In the area of reading, Ms. Smith confirmed that, although Johnny can generally read what he is given out loud and appears to be able to read material silently when given an assignment, reading appears effortful for him and that it is apparent by his answers to test questions that he has not always understood or remembered what he has read. Ms. Smith indicated that she feels Johnny would benefit greatly from some type of tutoring and/or speech-language therapy to help him address the difficulties discussed earlier.

IX. Classroom Observation

A classroom observation at Johnny's school could not be arranged due to time constraints (i.e., need to complete the evaluation by a certain timeline, before the end of the university semester). Assuming Johnny is enrolled for intervention at the _____ University Speech and Hearing Clinic, a classroom observation will be scheduled next semester, pending parental approval and approval from school administrators and classroom teachers at _____ Elementary school.

X. Diagnosis

Mild to moderate expressive language deficit; learning disability with accompanying reading and writing deficits (as confirmed by educational diagnostician).

XI. Recommendations

It is felt that Johnny would substantially benefit from speech-language intervention of a holistic literature-based nature (i.e., incorporating aspects of speaking, listening, reading, and writing into his individualized educational plan). The goal would be to reduce the significant gap between Johnny's receptive language abilities (which are somewhat above chronological age-expectancies) and his expressive language abilities (which are lower in comparison). If Johnny were to be seen at the _____ University Speech and Hearing Clinic for services (particularly in the After-School Language Literacy Clinic), efforts would be made to coordinate his intervention with his academic curricular needs and to consult with his parents and teachers and any other service providers at his school and/or at the Institute in order to develop an appropriate individualized treatment plan.

1. It is recommended that Ms. Doe and Johnny follow through with recommendations made by the educational diagnostician at the Institute with regard to his overall educational planning and intervention.

Continued

2. It is recommended that Johnny be seen at the After-School Language Literacy Program (part of the _____ University Speech and Hearing Clinic) for language-literacy based intervention, 1 to 2 hours per week starting in the Fall semester, to improve his oral and written language abilities. This intervention would be holistic in nature, focusing simultaneously on all language modalities (i.e., reading, writing, speaking, and listening). Intervention would be collaborative in nature, designed to coordinate with any other educational services Johnny might be receiving through the Institute and/or at his school. Parent training (i.e., allowing parents to watch sessions in order to learn some of the scaffolding, or cueing, strategies) to assist Johnny with his reading, writing, speaking, and listening abilities would also be an important part of the intervention format. Observation facilities at the _____ University Speech and Hearing Clinic would allow for this sort of parental training and involvement, which has proved to be extremely facilitative of client progress in the past.

_____

Speech-language pathologist

References

Aaron, P. G., Joshi, M., & Williams, K. (1999). Not all reading disabilities are alike. *Journal of Learning Disabilities, 32*(2), 120-137.

Americans with Disabilities Act, Public Law 101-336, signed into law July 26, 1990.

Anderson, E. S. (1975). Cups and glasses: Learning that boundaries are vague. *Journal of Child Language, 2,* 79-103.

Anderson, J. R. (1985). *Cognitive psychology and its implications* (2nd ed.). New York: W. H. Freeman.

Anderson, R. C. (1978). Schema directed processes in language comprehension. In A. Lesgold, J. Pelegrino, S. Fokhema, & R. Glaser (Eds.), *Cognitive psychology and instruction* (pp. 67-82). New York: Plenum Press.

Anderson, R. C., Reynolds, R. E., Schallert, D. I., & Goetz, E. T. (1977). Frameworks for comprehending discourse. *American Educational Research Journal, 14,* 367-382.

Anderson, R. C., Spiro, R. J., & Anderson, M. C. (1978). Schemata as scaffolding for the representation of information in connected discourse. *American Educational Research Journal, 15,* 433-440.

Anglin, J. M. (1993). Vocabulary development: A morphological analysis. *Monographs of the Society for Research in Child Development, 58*(10), 1-165.

Annett, M. (1985). *Left, right, hand and brain: The right shift theory.* London: Erlbaum.

Apel, K., & Masterson, J. J. (2001). Theory-guided spelling assessment and intervention: A case study. *Language, Speech, and Hearing Services in Schools, 32*(3), 182-195.

Apel, K., Masterson, J. J., Lombardino, L. J., Ahmed, S. T., Moats, L. C., Pollock, K., Templeton, S., & Bear, D. R. (2000). What is the role of the speech-language pathologist in assessing and facilitating spelling skills? *Topics in Language Disorders, 20*(3), 83-98.

Applebee, A. (1978). *The child's concept of story.* Chicago: University of Chicago Press.

Baddeley, A., Gathercole, S., & Papagno, C. (1998). The phonological loop as a language learning device. Psychological *Review, 105*(1), 158-173.

Badon, L. C. (1993). *Comparison of word recognition and story retelling under the conditions of contextualized versus decontextualized reading events in at-risk poor readers.* Unpublished doctoral dissertation, Louisiana State University, Baton Rouge.

Baker, L., & Brown, A. L. (1984). Metacognitive skills and reading. In P. D. Pearson (Ed.), *Handbook of reading research* (pp. 353-394). New York: Longman.

Barenbaum, E., Newcomer, P., & Nodine, B. (1987). Children's ability to write stories as a function of variation in task, age and developmental level. *Learning Disability Quarterly, 10,* 175-188.

Bartlett, F. C. (1932). *Remembering: A study in experimental and social psychology.* Cambridge, England: Cambridge University Press.

Beck, A. R., & Dennis, M. (1997). Speech-language pathologists' and teachers' perceptions of classroom-based interventions. *Language, Speech, and Hearing Services in Schools, 28,* 146-152.

Beck, I., & McKeown, M. (1981). Developing questions that promote comprehension: The story map. *Language Arts, 58*(8), 913-918.

Benelli, B., Arcuri, L., & Marchesini, G. (1988). Cognitive and linguistic factors in the development of word definitions. *Journal of Child Language, 15,* 619-635.

Berlyne, D. E. (1949). Interest as a psychological concept. *British Journal of Psychology, 39,* 184-195.

Berlyne, D. E. (1960). *Conflict, arousal, and curiosity.* New York: McGraw-Hill.

Bierwisch, M., & Kiefer, F. (1970). Remarks on definitions in natural language. In F. Kiefer (Ed.), *Studies in syntax and semantics* (pp. 55-79). Dordrecht, Germany: Reidel.

Bishop, D. V. M., & Adams, C. (1992). Comprehension problems in children with specific language impairment: Literal and inferential meaning. *Journal of Speech and Hearing Research, 35,* 119-129.

Bishop, D. V. M., & Edmundson, A. (1987). Language-impaired four-year olds: Distinguishing transient from persistent impairment. *Journal of Speech and Hearing Disorders, 52,* 156-173.

Block, F. K. (1995). Collaboration: Changing times. In D. F. Tibbits (Ed.), *Language intervention beyond the primary grades* (pp. 61-136). Austin, TX: Pro-Ed.

Bloom, P. (2000). *How children learn the meanings of words.* Cambridge, MA: MIT Press.

Blosser, J. L., & Kratcoski, A. (1997). PACs: A framework for determining appropriate service delivery options. *Language, Speech, and Hearing Services in Schools, 28,* 99-107.

Botting, N. (2002). Narrative as a tool for the assessment of linguistic and pragmatic impairments. *Child Language Teaching and Therapy, 18*(1), 1-21.

Bourassa, D. C., & Treiman, R. (2001). Spelling development and disability: The importance of linguistic factors. *Language, Speech, and Hearing Services in Schools, 32*(3), 172-81.

Bransford, J. D., Stein, B. S., Vye, N. J., Franks, J. J., Auble, P. M., Mezynski, K. J., & Perfetto, G. A. (1982). Differences in approaches to learning: An overview. *Journal of Experimental Psychology: General, 3,* 390-398.

Brown, A. (1975). The development of memory: Knowing, knowing about knowing, and knowing how to know. In H. W. Reese (Ed.), *Advances in child development and behavior.* New York: Academic Press.

Brown, G., & Yule, G. (1983). *Discourse analysis.* New York: Cambridge University Press.

Brown, K. J., Sinatra, G. M., & Wagstaff, J. M. (1996). Exploring the potential of analogy instruction to support children's spelling development. *Elementary School Journal, 97,* 81-99.

Bruner, J. (1986). *Actual minds, possible worlds.* Cambridge, MA: Harvard University Press.

Butler, K. (1999a). From oracy to literacy: Changing clinical perceptions. *Topics in Language Disorders, 20*(1), 14-32.

Butler, K. (1999b). From the editor. *Topics in Language Disorders, 20*(1), iv-v.

Campbell, T. F., & Bain, B. A. (1991). How long to treat: A multiple outcome approach. *Language, Speech, and Hearing Services in Schools, 22,* 271-276.

Carey, S. (1978). The child as word learner. In M. Halle, J. Bresnan, & G. Miller (Eds.), *Linguistic theory and psychological reality* (pp. 264-297). Cambridge, MA: MIT Press.

Carnine, D., Kameenui, E., & Woolfson, N. (1982). Training of textual dimension related to text-based inference. *Journal of Reading Behavior, 14,* 335-340.

Cazden, C. B. (1988). *Classroom discourse: The language of teaching and learning.* Portsmouth, NH: Heinemann.

Chall, J. (1987). Two vocabularies for reading: Recognition and meaning. In M. G. McKeown and M. E. Curtis (Eds.), *The nature of vocabulary acquisition* (pp. 7-18). Hillsdale, NJ: Erlbaum.

Chapman, M. (1994). The emergence of genres: Some findings from an examination of first-grade writing. *Written Communication, 11,* 348-380.

Chou-Hare, V., & Pulliam, C. A. (1980). Teacher questioning: A verification and an extension. *Journal of Reading Behavior, 12,* 69-72.

Cirrin, F. M., & Penner, S. G. (1995). Classroom-based and consultative service delivery models for language intervention. In M. E. Fey, J. Windsor, & S. F. Warren (Eds.), *Language intervention: Preschool through the elementary years* (Vol. 5, pp. 333-362). Baltimore: Paul H. Brookes.

Conti-Ramsden, G., & Adams, C. (1995). Transitions from the clinic to school: The changing picture of specific language impaired children from pre-school to school age. *Journal of Clinical Speech and Language Studies, 5,* 1-11.

Conti-Ramsden, G., & Botting, N. (1999). Classification of children with specific language impairment:

Longitudinal considerations. *Journal of Speech, Language, and Hearing Research, 42,* 1195-1204.

Conti-Ramsden, G., Crutchley, A., & Botting, N. (1997). The extent to which psychometric tests differentiate subgroups of children with SLI. *Journal of Speech, Language, and Hearing Research, 40,* 765-777.

Cook-Gumperz, J., & Gumperz, J. J. (1982). Communicating competence in educational perspective. In L. C. Wilkinson (Ed.), *Communicating in the classroom* (pp. 13-24). New York: Academic Press.

Cowley, J. (1996). *Jim's trumpet.* Bothell, WA: Wright Group.

Crais, E., & Chapman, R. (1987). Story recall and inferencing skills in language-learning disabled and nondisabled children. *Journal of Speech and Hearing Disorders, 52,* 50-55.

Damico, J. S. (1985). Clinical discourse analysis: A functional approach to language assessment. In C. Simon (Ed.), *Communication skills and classroom success: Assessment of language–learning disabled students* (pp. 165-193). London: Taylor & Francis.

Damico, J. S. (1988). The lack of efficacy in language therapy: A case study. *Language, Speech, and Hearing Services in Schools, 19,* 51-66.

Davey, B., & Macready, G. B. (1985). Prerequisite relations among inference tasks for good and poor readers. *Journal of Educational Psychology, 77,* 539-552.

Davis, Z. T., & McPherson, M. D. (1989). Story map instruction: A road map for reading comprehension. *The Reading Teacher, 43,* 232-240.

DeKemel, K. (1998). *Improving oral reading, inferencing, and narrative abilities in school-age children.* Unpublished doctoral dissertation, Louisiana State University, Baton Rouge.

DeKemel, K. (2002, April). *Managing the dismissal dilemma for school-age language-learning-disabled students.* Texas Speech-Language-Hearing Association Annual Convention.

DeKemel, K., & Ortego, J. (1994). *Using story maps to improve LLD children's oral and written narratives.* Paper presented at the Fourteenth Annual Superconference on Special Education, Baton Rouge, LA.

De La Touche, G. (1995). *Ali Baba.* Grandreams Limited, NY: Shooting Star Press.

Dodge, E. P. (1998). *Communication lab 1: A classroom communication program.* San Diego: Singular Publishing Group.

Dowhower, S. (1997). The method of repeated readings. *The Reading Teacher, 50*(5), 376-381.

Dyson, A. (1993). A sociocultural perspective on symbolic development in primary grade classrooms. In C. Daiute (Ed.), *The development of literacy through social interaction* (pp. 25-40). San Francisco: Jossey-Bass Publishers.

Ebert, K. A., & Prelock, P. A. (1994). Speech-language pathologists' perceptions of integrated service delivery in school settings. *Language, Speech, and Hearing Services in Schools, 25,* 258-267.

Ehren, B. J. (2000). Maintaining a therapeutic focus and sharing responsibility for student success: Keys to in-classroom speech-language services. *Language, Speech, and Hearing Services in Schools, 31,* 219-229.

Elksnin, L., & Capilouto, G. (1994). Speech-language pathologists' perceptions of integrated service delivery in school settings. *Language, Speech, and Hearing Services in Schools, 25,* 258-267.

Ellis-Weismer, S. (1985). Constructive comprehension abilities exhibited by language-disabled children. *Journal of Speech and Hearing Research, 28,* 175-184.

Ezell, M. C. (1995). *Evaluating the efficacy of communicative reading strategies with high risk first grade students.* Unpublished doctoral dissertation, Louisiana State University, Baton Rouge.

Foundas, A. L. (2001a). The neural basis of language: Current neuroimaging perspectives (Forward). *Topics in Language Disorders, 21*(3), vii.

Foundas, A. L. (2001b). The anatomical basis of language. *Topics in Language Disorders, 21*(3), 1-19.

Fox, B. J., & Wright, M. (1997). Connecting school and home literacy experiences through cross-age reading. *The Reading Teacher, 50*(5), 396-403.

Fraser, B. (1990). Perspectives on politeness. *Journal of Pragmatics, 14,* 219-236.

Galaburda, A. M., Sherman, G. F., Rosen, G. D., Aboitz, F., & Geschwind, N. (1985). Developmental dyslexia: Four consecutive patients with cortical anomalies. *Annals of Neurology, 18,* 222-233.

Gantwerk, B. (1985). Issues to address in criteria development. In *Caseload issues in schools: How to make better decisions* (pp. 43-45). Rockville, MD: American Speech-Language-Hearing Association.

Garfield, J. L. (1990). Convention, context, and meaning: Conditions on natural language understanding. In J. L. Garfield (Ed.), *Foundations of cognitive science: The essential readings.* New York: Paragon House.

Gauger, L. M., Lombardino, L. J., & Leonard, C. M. (1997). Brain morphology in children with specific language impairment. *Journal of Speech, Language, and Hearing Research, 40,* 1272-1284.

Geschwind, N., & Galaburda, A. (1985). Cerebral lateralization: Biological mechanisms, associations, and pathology I. A hypothesis and a program for research. *Archives of Neurology, 42,* 428-459.

Geschwind, N., & Levitsky, W. (1968). Human brain: Left-right asymmetries in temporal speech region. *Science, 161,* 186-187.

Gillam, R. B. (1989). An investigation of the oral language, reading, and written language competencies of language impaired and normally achieving school-age children. Doctoral dissertation, Indiana University. (University Microfilms, No. 9012207)

Gillam, R. B., & Johnston, J. R. (1992). Spoken and written language relationships in language/learning impaired and normally achieving school-age children. *Journal of Speech and Hearing Research, 35,* 1301-1315.

Goodman, K. S. (1965). A linguistic study of cues and miscues in reading. *Elementary English, 42,* 639-643.

Goodman, K. S. (1969). Analysis of oral reading miscues: Applied psycholinguistics. *Reading Research Quarterly, 1,* 9-30.

Goodman, K. S. (1984). Unity in reading. In A. C. Purves & O. Niles (Eds.), *Becoming readers in a complex society* (Part 1, pp. 79-114). Chicago: University of Chicago Press.

Goodman, K. S., & Gollasch, F. V. (1980). Word omissions: Deliberate and non-deliberate. *Reading Research Quarterly, 16,* 6-31.

Goodman, K. S., & Goodman, Y. M. (1977). Learning about psycholinguistic processes by analyzing oral reading. *Harvard Educational Review, 47,* 317-333.

Gordon, C., & Pearson, P. D. (1983). *Effects of instruction in meta-comprehension and inferencing on children's comprehension abilities* (Tech. Rep. No. 277). Urbana, IL: Center for the Study of Reading, University of Illinois.

Graesser, A. C., & Clark, L. C. (1985). *Structures and procedures of implicit knowledge.* Norwood, NJ: Ablex.

Graesser, A. C., Singer, M., & Trabasso, T. (1994). Constructing inferences during narrative text comprehension. *Psychological Review, 101*(3), 371-395.

Graham, S. (1997). Executive control in the revising of students with learning and writing disabilities. *Journal of Educational Psychology, 89,* 223-234.

Graham, S. (1999). Handwriting and spelling instruction for students with learning disabilities: A review. *Learning Disability Quarterly, 22,* 78-98.

Graham, S., & Harris, K. R. (1999). Assessment and intervention in overcoming writing difficulties: An illustration from the self-regulated strategy development model. *Language, Speech, and Hearing Services in Schools, 30*(3), 255-264.

Graham, S., Harris, K., & Loynachan, C. (1994). The spelling for writing list. *Journal of Learning Disability, 27,* 210-214.

Graham, S., Harris, K., & Loynachan, C. (1996). The directed spelling thinking activity: Application with high frequency words. *Learning Disabilities Research and Practice, 11,* 34-40.

Graybeal, C. M. (1981). Memory for stories in language-impaired children. *Applied Psycholinguistics, 2,* 269-283.

Green, J. L., Weade, R., & Graham, K. (1988). Lesson construction and student participation: A sociolinguistic analysis. In J. L. Green & J. P. Harker (Eds.), *Multiple perspective analysis of classroom discourse* (pp. 11-47). Norwood, NJ: Ablex.

Greenhalgh, K. S., & Strong, C. J. (2001). Literate language features in spoken narratives of children with typical language and children with language impairments. *Language, Speech, and Hearing Services in Schools, 32,* 114-125.

Grice, H. P. (1975). Logic and conversation. In P. Cole & J. L. Morgan (Eds.), *Syntax and semantics: Vol. 3. Speech acts* (pp. 41-58). New York: Academic Press.

Grice, H. P. (1989). *Studies in the way of words.* Cambridge, MA: Harvard University Press.

Guszak, F. J. (1967). Teacher questioning and reading. *The Reading Teacher, 21,* 227-234.

Hansen, J. (1981). The effects of inference training and practice on young children's comprehension. *Reading Research Quarterly, 16,* 391-417.

Hansen, J., & Pearson, P. D. (1983). An instructional study: Improving the inferential comprehension of good and poor fourth grade readers. *Journal of Educational Psychology, 75,* 821-829.

Harris, T. L., & Hodges, R. E. (1995). *The literacy dictionary: The vocabulary of reading and writing.* Newark, DE: International Reading Association.

Hebb, D. O. (1949). *The organization of behavior: A neuropsychological theory.* New York: Wiley.

Hernandez, S. N. (1989). *Effects of communicative reading strategies on the literacy behaviors of third grade poor readers.* Unpublished doctoral dissertation, Louisiana State University, Baton Rouge.

Hoggan, K. C., & Strong, C. J. (1994). The magic of "once upon a time": Narrative teaching strategies. *Language, Speech, and Hearing Services in Schools, 25,* 76-89.

Holmes, B. C. (1985). The effects of a strategy and sequenced materials on the inferential comprehension of disabled readers. *Journal of Learning Disabilities, 18,* 542-546.

Idol, L. (1987). Story mapping as a means of improving reading comprehension. *Learning Disability Quarterly 10* (3), 214-229.

Idol, L., & Croll, V. J. (1987). Story-mapping training as a means of improving reading comprehension. *Learning Disabilities Quarterly, 10,* 214-229.

Irwin, P. A., & Mitchell, J. N. (1983). A procedure for assessing the richness of retellings. *Journal of Reading, 26,* 394-395.

Joffe, B. S., & Doyle, J. (1996). The persisting communicative difficulties of "remediated" language-impaired children. *European Journal of Communication Disorders, 31,* 369-386.

Johnson, C. J., & Anglin, J. M. (1995). Qualitative developments in the content and form of children's definitions. *Journal of Speech-Language-Hearing Research, 38,* 612-629.

Johnson, D. (1987). Disorders of written language. In D. Johnson & J. Blalock (Eds.), *Adults with learning disabilities: Clinical studies* (pp. 173-204). New York: Grune & Stratton.

Just, M. A., & Carpenter, P. A. (1992). A capacity theory of comprehension: Individual differences in working memory. *Psychological Review, 99,* 122-149.

Kaderavek, J. N., & Sulzby, E. (2000). Narrative production by children with and without specific language impairment: Oral narratives and emergent readings. *Journal of Speech, Language and Hearing Research, 43,* 34-49.

Kamhi, A. G., & Catts, H. W. (1991). *Reading disabilities: A developmental language perspective.* Boston: Allyn & Bacon.

Kamhi, A. G., & Hinton, L. N. (2000). Explaining individual differences in spelling ability. *Topics in Language Disorders, 20*(3), 37-49.

Kamil, M. I. (1984). Current traditions in reading research. In P. D. Pearson (Ed.), *Handbook of reading research* (pp. 39-62). New York: Longman.

Kapur, S., Craik, F., Jones, C., Brown, G., Houle, S., & Tulving, E. (1995). Functional role of the prefrontal cortex in retrieval of memories: A PET study. *Neuroreport, 6,* 1880-1884.

Kass, A. (1992). Question asking, artificial intelligence, and human creativity. In T. W. Lauer, E. Peacock, & A. C. Graesser (Eds.), *Question and information processing.* Hillsdale, NJ: Erlbaum.

Kintsch, W. (1980). Learning from text, levels of comprehension: A constructive integration model. *Psychological Review, 95,* 163-182.

Kintsch, W. (1988). The role of knowledge in discourse comprehension construction-integration model. *Psychological Review, 95,* 163-182.

Kintsch, W. (1992). A cognitive architecture for comprehension. In H. L. Pick, P. van den Broek, & D. C. Knill (Eds.), *The study of cognition: Conceptual and methodological issues* (pp. 143-164). Washington, DC: American Psychological Association.

Kintsch, W., & van Dijk, T. A. (1978). Toward a model of text comprehension and production. *Psychological Review, 85*(5):363-394.

Klein, D. E., & Murphy, G. L. (2001). The representation of polysemous words. *Journal of Memory and Language, 45,* 259-282.

Kletzien, S. B. (1991). Strategy use by good and poor comprehenders reading expository text of differing levels. *Reading Research Quarterly, 26,* 67-86.

Kos, R. (1991). Persistence of reading disabilities: The voices of four middle school students. *American Educational Research Journal, 28,* 875-895.

Koskinen, P. S., Gambrell, L. B., & Kapinus, B. A. (1993). The use of retellings for portfolio assessment of reading comprehension. In J. F. Almasi (Ed.), *Literacy: Issues and practices* (Vol. 10, pp. 41-77). Silver Spring, MD: State of Maryland International Reading Association Yearbook.

Kroll, R. M., & De Nil, L. F. (1998). Positron emission tomography studies of stuttering: Their relationship to our theoretical and clinical understanding of the disorder. *Journal of Speech Language Pathology and Audiology, 22*(4), 261-270.

LaBerge, D., & Samuels, S. J. (1974). Toward a theory of automatic information processing in reading. *Cognitive Psychology, 6,* 293-323.

Lakoff, R. (1973). The logic of politeness: Or, minding your p's and q's. In C. Corum, T. C. Smith-Stark, A. Weiser (Eds.), *Papers from the Ninth Regional Meeting of the Chicago Linguistic Society* (pp. 292-305). Chicago: Chicago Linguistic Society.

Lane, A. G., Foundas, A. L., & Leonard, C. M. (2001). The evolution of neuroimaging research and developmental language disorders. *Topics in Language Disorders, 21*(3), 20-41.

Leech, G. N. (1983). *Principles of pragmatics.* London: Longman.

Lehnert, W., Dyer, M. G., Johnson, P., Yang, C., & Harley, S. (1983). BORIS: An experiment in in-depth understanding of narratives. *Artificial Intelligence, 20*(1), 15-62.

Leonard, C. M., Voeller, K. S., Lombardino, L. J., Morris, M. K., Hynd, G. W., Alexander, A. W., Anderson, H. G., Garofalakis, M., Honeyman, J. C., Mao, J., Agee, F., & Staab, E. V. (1993). Anomalous cerebral structure in dyslexia revealed in MRI. *Archives of Neurology, 50,* 461-469.

Liles, B. Z. (1985). Cohesion in the narratives of normal and language-disordered children. *Journal of Speech and Hearing Research, 28,* 123-133.

Liles, B. Z. (1987). Episode organization and cohesive conjunctives in narratives of children with and without language disorder. *Journal of Speech & Hearing Research, 30,* 185-196.

Liles, B. Z. (1993). Narrative discourse in children with language disorders and children with normal language: A critical review of the literature. *Journal of Speech and Hearing Research, 36,* 868-882.

Lindblom, K. (2001). Cooperating with Grice: A cross disciplinary metaperspective on uses of Grice's cooperative principle. *Journal of Pragmatics, 33,* 1601-1623.

Lipson, M. Y., & Wixson, K. K. (1986). Reading disability research: An interactionist perspective. *Review of Educational Research, 56,* 111-136.

Litowitz, B. (1977). Learning to make definitions. *Journal of Child Language, 4,* 289-304.

Luria, A. R. (1966). *Higher cortical functions in man.* New York: Basic Books.

MacLean, I. (2000). *Effects of interactive vocabulary instruction on reading comprehension of students with learning disabilities: Action research report.* Bellingham, WA: Western Washington University, Woodring College of Education.

Mandler, J. M., & Johnson, N. S. (1977). Remembrance of things past: Story structure and recall. *Cognitive Psychology, 9,* 111-151.

Markowitz, J., & Franz, S. (1988). The development of defining style. *International Journal of Lexicography, 1*(3), 253-267.

Masterson, J. J., & Apel, K. (2000). Spelling assessment: Charting a path to optimal intervention. *Topics in Language Disorders, 20*(3), 50-65,

Masterson, J. J., & Crede, L. A. (1999). Learning to spell: Implications for assessment and intervention. *Language, Speech, and Hearing Services in Schools, 30*(3), 243-254.

McCormick, S. (1992). Disabled readers' erroneous responses to inferential comprehension questions: Description and analysis. *Reading Research Quarterly, 27,* 55-77.

McGhee-Bidlack, B. (1991). The development of noun definitions: A metalinguistic analysis. *Journal of Child Language, 18,* 417-434.

McGregor, K. K., Friedman, R. M., Reilly, R. M., & Newman, R. M. (2002). Semantic representation in young children. *Journal of Speech, Language, and Hearing Research, 45,* 332-346.

Mehan, H. (1979). *Learning lessons: Social organization in the classroom.* Cambridge, MA: Harvard University Press.

Merritt, D. D., & Liles, B. Z. (1987). Story grammar ability in children with and without language disorder: Story generation, story retelling, and story comprehension. *Journal of Speech and Hearing Research, 30,* 539-552.

Merritt, D. D., & Liles, B. Z. (1989). Narrative analysis: Clinical applications of story generation and story retelling. *Journal of Speech and Hearing Disorders, 54,* 429-438.

Miller, G. A., & Gildea, P. M. (1987). How children learn words. *Scientific American, 257,* 94-99.

Miller, L. (1989). Classroom-based language intervention. *Language, Speech, and Hearing Services in Schools, 20,* 153-169.

Montague, M., Maddux, C. D., & Dereshiwsky, M. (1990). Story grammar and comprehension and production of narrative prose by students with learning disabilities. *Journal of Learning Disabilities, 23,* 190-197.

Moscovitch, M. (1994). Memory and working with memory: Evaluation of a component process model and comparisons with other models. In D. L. Schacter & E. Tulving (Eds.), *Memory systems* (pp. 269-310). Cambridge, MA: MIT/Bradford Press.

Moss, B. (1997). Richness of retelling scale. *Reading Research and Instruction, 37*(1), 1-13.

Nagy, W., & Anderson, R. (1984). How many words are there in printed school English? *Reading Research Quarterly, 19,* 304-330.

Nelson, K. (1985). *Making sense: The acquisition of shared meaning.* New York: Academic Press.

Nelson, K. (1986). *Event knowledge: Structure and function in development.* Hillsdale, NJ: Erlbaum.

Nelson, K. (1991). Event knowledge and the development of language functions. In J. Miller (Ed.), *Research on child language disorders: A decade of progress* (pp. 125-142). Austin, TX: Pro-Ed.

Nelson, N. W. (1989). Curriculum-based language assessment and intervention. *Language, speech and hearing services in schools, 20,* 170-184.

Nicholas, D. W., & Trabasso, T. (1980). Toward a taxonomy of inferences for story comprehension. In F. Wilkening, J. Becker, & T. Trabasso (Eds.), *Information integration in children.* Hillsdale, NJ: Erlbaum.

Norris, J. (1988). Using communication strategies to enhance reading acquisition. *The Reading Teacher, 41,* 368-373.

Norris, J. (1989). Providing language remediation in the classroom: An integrated language-to-reading intervention method. *Language, Speech, and Hearing Services in Schools, 20,* 205-219.

Norris, J. (1991). From frog to prince: Using written language as a context for language learning. *Topics in Language Disorders, 12*(1), 1-6.

Norris, J. (1992). Some questions and answers about whole language. *American Journal of Speech-Language Pathology and Audiology, 1*(4), 11-14.

Norris, J., & Hoffman, P. (1993). *Whole language intervention for school-age children.* San Diego: Singular Publishing Group.

Olivier, C., Hecker, L., Klucken, J., & Westby, C. (2000). Language: The embedded curriculum in postsecondary education. *Topics in Language Disorders, 21*(1), 15-29.

Owens, R. (1991). Narrative analysis. In *Language disorders: A functional approach to assessment and intervention.* Columbus, OH: Macmillan.

Owens, R. (1996). *Language development: An introduction* (4th ed.). Boston: Allyn & Bacon.

Owens, R. (1999). *Language disorders: A functional approach to assessment and intervention* (3rd ed.). Boston: Allyn & Bacon.

Palmer, W. S. (1982). *An observational study in secondary English classrooms.* Paper presented at the National Reading Conference, Clearwater, FL.

Paris, S. G., & Lindauer, B. K. (1976). The role of inference in children's comprehension and memory for sentences. *Cognitive Psychology, 8,* 217-227.

Paris, S. G., Wasik, B. A., & Turner, J. C. (1991). The development of strategic readers. In R. Barr, M. L. Kamil, P. Mosenthal, & P. D. Pearson (Eds.), *Handbook of reading research* (Vol. II, pp. 609-640). New York: Longman.

Parkins, E. J. (1990). Psychological development: An integrated description. In E. J. Parkins (Ed.), *Equilibration, mind, and brain: Toward an integrated psychology.* New York: Praeger.

Paul, R. (1989). *Profiles of toddlers with delayed expressive language development.* Paper presented at the Biannual Meeting of the Society for Research in Child Development, Kansas City, MO.

Paul, R. (1993). Outcomes of early expressive language delay. *Journal of Childhood Communication Disorders, 15,* 7-14.

Paul, R. (1996). Clinical implications of the natural history of slow expressive language development. *American Journal of Speech-Language Pathology, 5*(2), 5-22.

Pearson, P. D., Hansen, J., & Gordon, C. (1979). The effect of background knowledge on young children's comprehension of explicit and implicit information. *Journal of Reading Behavior, 11,* 201-209.

Piaget, J. (1952). *The origins of intelligence.* New York: International Universities Press.

Piaget, J. (1954). *The construction of reality in the child.* New York: Basic Books.

Piaget, J. (1960). *The child's conception of physical causality.* Paterson, NJ: Littlefield, Adams.

Pinker, S. (1982). A theory of the acquisition of lexical interpretive grammars. In J. Bresnan (Ed.), *The mental representation of grammatical relations.* Cambridge, MA: MIT Press.

Plante, E. (1991). MRI findings in the parents and siblings of specifically language-impaired boys. *Brain and Language, 41,* 67-80.

Plante, E., Swisher, L., Vance, R., & Rapcsak, S. (1991). MRI findings in boy with specific language impairment. *Brain and Language, 41,* 52-66.

Preis, S., Jancke, L., Schittler, P., Huang, Y., & Steinmetz, H. (1998). Normal intrasylvian anatomical asymmetry in children with developmental language disorder. *Neuropsychology, 36*(9), 849-855.

Prelock, P. A. (2000). Multiple perspectives for determining the roles of speech-language pathologists in inclusionary classrooms. *Language, Speech, and Hearing Services in Schools, 31,* 213-218.

Purcell, S., & Liles, B. Z. (1992). Cohesion repairs in the narratives of normal-language and language-disordered school-age children. *Journal of Speech and Hearing Research, 35,* 354-362.

Rescorla, L. (1989). The Language Development Survey: A screening tool for delayed language in toddlers. *Journal of Speech and Hearing Disorders, 54,* 587-599.

Rescorla, L. (1990, June). *Outcomes of expressive language delay.* Paper presented at the Symposium for Research in Child Language Disorders, Madison, WI.

Reutzel, D. R. (1984). Story mapping: An alternative approach to comprehension. *Reading World, 24,* 16-25.

Roth, F. P. (2000). Narrative writing: Development and teaching children with writing difficulties. *Topics in Language Disorders, 20*(4), 15-28.

Roth, F. P., & Spekman, N. J. (1986). Narrative discourse: Spontaneously generated stories of learning-disabled and normally achieving students. *Journal of Speech and Hearing Disorders, 51,* 8-23.

Rumelhart, D. E. (1975). Notes on a schema for stories. In D. G. Bobrow & A. Collins (Eds.), *Representation and understanding: Studies in cognitive science.* New York: Academic Press.

Rupley, W., Logan, J., & Nichols, W. (1999). Vocabulary instruction in a balanced reading program. *The Reading Teacher, 52,* 336-346.

Sadker, M., & Sadker, D. (1982). *Sex equity handbook for schools.* New York: Longman.

Samuels, S. J. (1976). Automatic decoding and reading comprehension. *Language Arts, 53,* 323-325.

Samuels, S. J., & Kamil, M. L. (1984). Models of reading process. In P. D. Pearson (Ed.), *Handbook of reading research* (pp. 185-224). New York: Longman.

Schacter, D. (1996). *Searching for memory: The brain, the mind, and the past.* New York: Basic Books.

Schank, R., & Abelson, R. (1977). *Scripts, plans, goals, and understanding: An inquiry into human knowledge structure.* Hillsdale, NJ: Erlbaum.

Schneider, P. (1996). Effects of pictures versus orally presented stories on story retellings by children with language impairment. *American Journal of Speech-Language Pathology, 5,* 86-96.

Scott, C. (1989). Problem writers: Nature, assessment, and intervention. In A. Kamhi & H. Catts (Eds.), *Reading disabilities: A developmental language perspective.* San Diego: College Hill.

Scott, C. (1999). Learning to write. In H. W. Catts & A. G. Kamhi (Eds.), *Language and reading disabilities* (pp. 224-258). Boston: Allyn & Bacon.

Scott, C. (2000). Principles and methods of spelling instruction: Applications for poor spellers. *Topics in Language Disorders, 20*(3), 66-82.

Scott, C., & Windsor, J. (2000). General language performance measures in spoken and written narrative and expository discourse of school-age children with language-learning disabilities. *Journal of Speech, Language, and Hearing Research, 43,* 324-339.

Semon, R. W. (1921). *The mneme.* London: Allen & Unwin. (Original work published 1904)

Semon, R. W. (1923). *Mnemic psychology* (B. Duffy, Trans.). London: Allen & Unwin. (Original work published 1909)

Singer, B. D., & Bashir, A. S. (1999). What are executive functions and self-regulation and what do they have to do with language-learning disorders? *Language, Speech, and Hearing Services in Schools, 30*(3), 265-273.

Slater, W. H. (1988). Current theory and research on what constitutes readable expository text. *The Technical Writing Teacher, XV*(3), 195-206.

Snow, C. E. (1990). The development of definitional skill. *Journal of Child Language, 17,* 697-710.

Spiro, R. J. (1980). Constructive processes in prose comprehension and recall. In R. J. Spiro, B. C. Bruce, & W. F. Brewer (Eds.), *Theoretical issues in reading comprehension: Perspectives from cognitive psychology, linguistics, artificial intelligence, and education* (pp. 245-278). Hillsdale, NJ: Erlbaum.

Spiro, R. J., & Myers, A. (1984). Individual differences and underlying cognitive processes in reading. In P. D. Pearson (Ed.), *Handbook of reading research* (pp. 471-501). New York: Longman.

Stahl, S. A., & Fairbanks, M. M. (1986). The effects of vocabulary instruction: A model-based meta-analysis. *Review of Educational Research, 56,* 72-110.

Stein, N. L., & Glenn, C. G. (1979). An analysis of story comprehension in elementary school children. In R. O. Freedle (Ed.), *New directions in discourse processing* (Vol. 2, pp. 53-120). Norwood, NJ: Ablex.

Stein, N. L., & Trabasso, T. (1985). The search after meaning: Comprehension and comprehension monitoring. In F. J. Morrison, C. Lord, & D. Keating (Eds.), *Applied developmental psychology* (Vol. 2, pp. 33-58). San Diego: Academic Press.

Sternberg, R. (1987). Most vocabulary is learned from context. In M. McKeown & M. Curtis (Eds.), *The nature of vocabulary acquisition* (pp. 89-106). Hillsdale, NJ: Erlbaum.

Stothard, S. E., Snowling, M. J., Bishop, D. V. M., Chipchase, B. B., & Kaplan, C. A. (1998). Language-impaired preschoolers: A follow-up into adolescence. *Journal of Speech, Language, and Hearing Research, 41,* 407-418.

Sturm, J. M., & Nelson, N. W. (1997). Formal classroom lesson: New perspectives on a familiar discourse event. *Language, Speech, and Hearing Services in Schools, 28,* 255-273.

Sulzby, E. (1996). Roles of oral and written language as children approach conventional literacy. In C. Pontecorvo, M. Orsolino, B. Burge, & L. B. Resnick (Eds.), *Children's early text construction* (pp. 25-46). Mahwah, NJ: Erlbaum.

Thorndyke, P. W. (1977). Cognitive structures in comprehension and memory of narrative discourse. *Cognitive Psychology, 9,* 77-110.

Throneburg, R. N., Calvert, L. K., Sturm, J. J., Paramboukas, A. A., & Paul, P. J. (2000). A comparison of service delivery models: Effects on curricular vocabulary skills in the school setting. *American Journal of Speech-Language Pathology, 9*(1), 10-20.

Tierney, R. J., & Pearson, P. D. (1981). Learning to learn from text: A framework for improving classroom practices. In E. Dishner, J. Readence, & T. Bean (Eds.), *Reading in the content area: Improving classroom instruction* (pp. 50-65). Dubuque, IA: Kendall Hunt.

Trabasso, T. (1981). On the making of inferences during reading and their assessment. In J. Guthrie (Ed.), *Comprehension and teaching: Research reviews* (pp. 56-76). Newark, DE: International Reading Association.

Trabasso, T., & Nicholas, D. W. (1980). Memory and inferences in the comprehension of narratives. In F. Wilkening, J. Becker, & T. Trabasso (Eds.), *Information integration by children* (pp. 215-242). Hillsdale, NJ: Erlbaum.

Treiman, R., & Bourassa, D. C. (2000). The development of spelling skill. *Topics in Language Disorders, 20*(3), 1-18.

Wallach, G., & Miller, L. (1988). Inference and cohesion. In *Language intervention and academic success.* San Diego: College Hill.

Watson, R. (1985). Towards a theory of definition. *Journal of Child Language, 12,* 181-197.

Weaver, C. A., & Kintsch, W. (1983). Expository text. In R. Barr, M. L. Kamil, P. B. Mosenthal, & P. D. Pearson (Eds.), *Handbook of reading research* (Vol. II, pp. 230-245). New York: Longman.

Webster's ninth new collegiate dictionary. (1990). Springfield, MA: Merriam-Webster.

Wehren, A., DeLisi, R., & Arnold, M. (1981). The development of noun definition. *Journal of Child Language, 8,* 165-175.

Wennerstrom, A. (2001). Intonation and evaluation in oral narratives. *Journal of Pragmatics, 33,* 1183-1206.

Westby, C. (1984). Development of narrative abilities. In G. P. Wallach & K. G. Butler (Eds.), *Language-learning disabilities in school-age children.* Baltimore: Williams & Wilkins.

Westby, C. (1997). There's more to passing than knowing the answers. *Language, Speech, and Hearing Services in Schools, 28,* 274-287.

Westby, C. E., & Clauser, P. S. (1999). The right stuff for writing: Assessing and facilitating written language. In H. W. Catts & A. G. Kamhi (Eds.), *Language and reading disabilities* (pp. 259-316). Boston: Allyn & Bacon.

Westby, C., & Farmer, S. S. (2000). Assessment and intervention with adults with LLD: A paradigm shift. *Topics in Language Disorders, 21*(1), vi-viii.

Will, M. (1986). *Educating students with learning problems: A shared responsibility.* Washington, DC: U.S. Office of Education, Office of Special Education and Rehabilitative Services.

Wilson, M. M . (1979). The processing strategies of average and below average readers answering factual and inferential questions on three equivalent passages. *Journal of Reading Behavior, 11,* 235-245.

Winne, P. H., Graham, L., & Prock, L. (1993). A model of poor readers' text-based inferencing: Effects of explanatory feedback. *Reading Research Quarterly, 28*(1), 53-66.

Wong, B. (1980). Activating the inactive learner: Use of questions/prompts to enhance comprehension and retention of implied information in learning-disabled children. *Learning Disability Quarterly, 3,* 29-37.

Wong, B. Y. L. (2000). Writing strategies instruction for expository essays for adolescents with and without learning disabilities. *Topics in Language Disorders, 20*(4), 29-44.

Wright, H. H., & Newhoff, M. (2001). Narration abilities of children with language-learning disabilities in response to oral and written stimuli. *American Journal of Speech-Language Pathology, 10,* 308-319.

Index